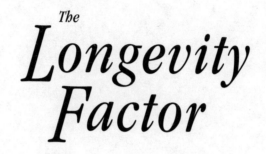

The
Longevity Factor

The
Longevity
Factor

How Resveratrol and Red Wine Activate
Genes for a Longer and Healthier Life

Joseph Maroon, MD

ATRIA BOOKS
NEW YORK • LONDON • TORONTO • SYDNEY

ATRIA BOOKS
A Division of Simon & Schuster, Inc.
1230 Avenue of the Americas
New York, NY 10020

Copyright © 2009 by Maroon Enterprises

All rights reserved, including the right to reproduce this book or portions thereof in any form whatsoever. For information address Atria Books Subsidiary Rights Department, 1230 Avenue of the Americas, New York, NY 10020

First Atria Books hardcover edition January 2009

ATRIA BOOKS and colophon are trademarks of Simon & Schuster, Inc.

For information about special discounts for bulk purchases, please contact Simon & Schuster Special Sales at 1-800-456-6798 or business@simonandschuster.com

Designed by Paul Dippolito

Manufactured in the United States of America

10 9 8 7 6 5 4 3 2 1

Library of Congress Cataloging-in-Publication Data
Maroon, Joseph C.
   The longevity factor: how resveratrol and red wine activate genes for a longer and healthier life / Joseph Maroon.
      p. cm.
   Includes bibliographical references and index.   1. Longevity.
2. Resveratrol—Health aspects.   I. Title.

RA776.75.M363 2009
613.2—dc2   2008042777

ISBN-13: 978-1-4165-5107-2
ISBN-10:   1-4165-5107-7

To

David Sinclair and Sandra Luikenhuis,
and to
Madeline, Natalie, and Benjamin—
the present and future of
research in living longer, healthier, and better

Contents

PART IV: UNLOCKING THE GENETIC SECRETS TO LIVING HEALTHIER AND LONGER

Foreword

For millennia, human beings have sought to enjoy longer, healthier lives. In some respects we have been quite successful; in the past two centuries, modern medicine succeeded in doubling the average life span—at least for those of us who live in industrialized nations. However, even the luckiest of us cannot expect to live much beyond 100 years, a limit that has changed very little throughout recorded history. The failure of any human, by chance or through various antiaging schemes, to exceed the 122-year record set by Frenchwoman Jeanne Calment on her death in 1997 has led many to conclude that nature has already reached the outer limit of the human life span. Cell biology, however, indicates something quite different. Many biologists are coming to believe that human beings have not been optimized for long life at all, and the true potential of the human form to endure when damage is prevented or repaired is unknown. In other words, our potential for longevity may be largely untapped.

Recognizing the potential for longer life and bringing it about, however, are two very different things. The quest for longevity has been full of surprises. For instance, aging is such a vastly complex biological process that the idea that it could be altered by something as simple as calorie reduction once seemed laughable. The notion gained traction, however, as its evolutionary benefits became clear, and then became widely accepted with the now seventy-five-year-old observation that rodents fed approximately 60 percent of the calories they desired outlived their healthy, well-fed counterparts by more than 50 percent in some cases.

The effort to identify and understand the genes controlling longevity, and to harness their power to improve the quality of human life, is a tremendously exciting and active area of scientific research. In this book Joe Maroon takes readers on a fascinating journey through some of the most recent and startling developments in this field. Chief among these is the emergence of a theory that genes capable of extending longevity may be kicked into action by specific plant-derived molecules in the human diet. Termed the "xenohormesis hypothesis," this theory may offer us a straightforward and safe way to activate and enhance our own evolutionary defenses against the ravages of age.

As a medical expert and skilled writer, Dr. Maroon possesses a unique ability to transport us seamlessly from the depths of molecular biology to the triumphs and limitations of modern medicine, and to make the latest findings and predictions accessible to the lay reader. Interweaving the stories of scientists and entrepreneurs with his own clinical experiences, Dr. Maroon has created a manuscript that is by turns informative, compelling, deeply personal, and, ultimately, inspiring.

Joseph A. Baur, PhD
Paul F. Glenn Laboratories for the
Biological Mechanisms of Aging, Harvard University

Introduction

In November 2006 headlines around the world blared the news of a series of scientific breakthroughs reported by such authoritative sources as Harvard Medical School, the National Institute on Aging (NIA)—part of the National Institutes of Health—and the Institute of Genetics and Molecular and Cellular Biology (IGBMC) in France. Could it really be possible that natural substances found in red wine could extend life, avert cancer and heart disease, help people maintain or even lose weight despite a high-fat diet, and create the muscles of a champion athlete without training? All these extraordinary effects were being observed in laboratory animals, offering reason to believe the same would hold true for humans. A new fountain of youth? Scientists at Harvard Medical School saw this as a distinct possibility.

Although I am a senior neurosurgeon and have published many papers and books in my own scientific field, I was totally unaware of this longevity research until a year before it became big news. In October 2005, while attending a neurosurgical meeting in Boston, I sat in on a lecture by Dr. David Sinclair, a brilliant evolutionary biologist, molecular geneticist, and director of the Paul F. Glenn Laboratories for the Biological Mechanisms of Aging at Harvard Medical School. At international medical meetings like this one, guest lecturers from other disciplines are frequently invited to share their work with the hope that cross-disciplinary work might emerge. I never could have guessed just how much this one lecture would completely change every aspect of my life.

A boyish, soft-spoken thirty-six-year-old former windsurfer from

Australia, Dr. Sinclair had chosen to address our group on the topic of "How to Activate Longevity Genes to Increase Strength, Endurance, and Prevent Neurodegenerative Diseases (like Alzheimer's)." His lecture described his research leading to the 2002 discovery of natural substances in red wine grapes and other plants that have the power to increase life span, fight disease, and change fat mice into rodent versions of Lance Armstrong. In Sinclair's lab at Harvard, mice on a high-fat, high-calorie diet were given *resveratrol,* a substance found in red wine grape skins. Sinclair discovered that resveratrol molecules from a plant source could activate certain animal-cell genetic pathways, owing to their small size and specialized shape, and once inside could produce amazing benefits. These included:

- Increased memory, as tested in mazes
- Reduced fat cells—despite a high-calorie diet
- Boosted energy and endurance in muscle cells
- Enhanced muscle strength and decreased fatigue
- Improved coordination and mobility
- Transformation of ordinary muscle fibers into the "slow" type found in well-trained athletes

But most remarkably, this class of molecule, which I will later refer to as a xeno factor, was also found to reduce the incidence of certain cancers, vascular disease, and brain degeneration, and prolonged the lives of treated mice by 25 percent.

These astounding observations showed that natural compounds from food could have a preventive effect on the most pressing health problems in the world and also significantly prolong life. Was it also possible that obesity, diabetes, heart attacks, cancer, degenerative disease of the brain, and other human debilitating diseases and conditions could also be markedly reduced using this natural food product effective in mice? And could human life also be extended simply by what we choose to eat? Sitting in the audience at David Sinclair's lecture, I was stunned. What did this mean? How might this change not just our own lives, but also the society we live in—and perhaps the entire world?

One year after this lecture, David Sinclair and his colleague Joseph Baur published their findings in *Nature,* one of the most prestigious scientific journals. (This was the paper that led to the international headlines I mentioned earlier.) Sinclair and Baur's work, along with that of many other scientists around the world, has provided the basis for a revolutionary new scientific approach to aging and its related diseases.

The groundwork for these revolutionary discoveries dates back to the 1930s, when scientists at Cornell University discovered that rodents placed on a near-starvation diet (60 percent of normal caloric intake) lived up to 50 percent longer, maintained youthful activity levels and appearance, and showed delays in age-related diseases. Later confirmed in other species, calorie restriction became the only known way to increase longevity. For the next sixty years, scientists tried to understand why. Just what happens on a molecular and biological level with caloric restriction to enhance longevity and health?

Finally, in the late 1980s to mid-1990s, researchers at the University of California's Irvine and San Francisco campuses and at the Massachusetts Institute of Technology (MIT) made a series of breakthroughs. They found specific sets of genes in laboratory animals that kept cells from wearing out, from being overwhelmed by free radicals, or from just "cashing in" after the reproductive phase. For the first time, it became clear that a single gene could alter the rate of aging, and that such a gene could be activated by caloric restriction or other stresses. These same genes exist in human beings and have become known as "survival" or "scarcity" genes.

Unfortunately, this near-starvation diet—despite its dramatic benefits—is intolerable for most people. I tried it for a month and decided the extra years weren't worth it! This makes even more exciting the recent discovery that substances like the small molecules found in red wine grape skins can activate these survival genes—without caloric restriction.

The secret of these natural compounds may actually be traced back to the grassy plains of Africa three or four million years ago. This was the time when we swung down from our tree habitats, walked upright as bipeds, began using tools, and gradually evolved into present-day *Homo sapiens*. When our ancestors were exposed to severe stress from environmental and climatic changes on the savanna, specific human genes would be activated that controlled carbohydrate, protein, and fat metabolism in order to improve their chances of survival. In times of plenty, our bodies typically burn food carbohydrates for energy and store food energy in the form of fat; during food shortages, these special genes mobilize this stored fat to survive. Exactly how external stresses like lack of food are communicated to our genes has been the subject of intense debate for decades. Now Drs. Sinclair and Baur and their associates at Harvard, Dr. Leonard Guarente and his associates at MIT, and other top scientists appear to have discovered a link.

Coexisting with our ancestors on the African savanna were plants that recognized and responded to environmental stresses such as drought, infection, pests, and harsh sun—just as humans did. To survive, these stressed plants activated their own survival genes, producing natural molecules to increase their own cellular defenses and repair mechanisms. For both primates and plants, Nietzsche's dictum "That which does not destroy me strengthens me" was playing out at the genetic level.

The remarkable development that Sinclair, Baur, and other scientists observed was the relationship between certain plant-produced molecules and the animals that eat them. We now have evidence that animals and humans can actually activate their own survival genes by ingesting specific molecules from plants that have been under stress. The plant molecules that they found in red wine grape skins (resveratrol) are produced by stress. In red grapes, and also certain other plants, these molecules are produced for the unique task of fighting off fungal infections and other invaders that might otherwise kill the plant. Laboratory mice that consumed these plant molecules also benefited from this same stress response. In other words, when ingested, plants "communicate" with animals and people, using the language of molecular genetics and activating the so-called survival genes. Although it may not be fully intentional, animals over millennia have learned to take advantage of this plant-based warning system.

The amazing task of mapping the system of human genes, which was completed by the Human Genome Project in 2001, has allowed scientists to study this plant-animal communication on an unprecedented level. The result is a new scientific field called *nutrigenomics,* which seeks to explain how nutritional substances, from blueberries to French fries, activate our genes for better and for worse.

This revolutionary branch of biology explains how substances from other species (*xeno*)—in this case, plants that have triggered their own protective response due to environmental stress (*hormesis*)—"talk" to people, stimulating human genes to set in motion similar cellular activities to promote survival. *Xenohormesis* holds the incredibly exciting promise of increasing mankind's longevity and reducing the effects of major killers like cancer, heart disease, and stroke—while keeping us thin! "That's why I don't think there is anything more important than this quest," Sinclair said. "That's why I take chances, and why the controversy is worth it: because I think we are right." Recently, as new research confirmed his hopes, he added, "We've found a gatekeeper of cell survival and potentially of the aging process itself."

One week after attending Dr. Sinclair's lecture, I traveled to Boston to visit him and Dr. Baur in their laboratory. Sinclair graciously showed me his lab while we discussed his plans for turbocharging his longevity molecules with techniques discovered by a fellow Australian, Peter Voigt. An engineer who specializes in extraction technology, Voigt lives in the center of the wine-growing Mornington Peninsula, south of Melbourne. After a number of tries, he found an ingenious way to superconcentrate stressed grape skin molecules, thereby amplifying their potential benefits for disease prevention and increased longevity.

David Sinclair and I discussed the possibility of creating specific human studies using Peter Voigt's "Australian extract," to see if humans would react to xenohormetic compounds, or *xeno factors,* the way animals did: with increased strength, endurance, memory, and coordination, and body weight stabilization. Indeed, the first study completed in 2007 was successful. It confirmed improvement in memory and endurance in humans similar to that observed in laboratory animals.

In this book I will recount the remarkable story of the brilliant scientists who discovered the human survival genes and cracked the longevity code—how these genes are activated and produce their powerful effect on weight, memory, hormones, and various organ systems. In addition, I will describe how Harvard scientists used sophisticated molecular gene tests to discover a total of nineteen xeno factors, which literally turn on longevity genes in animals.

I will also describe many of the research studies currently under way around the world that are exploring the use of these natural compounds for the prevention and treatment of diabetes, cancer, and heart disease in people. Since these molecules also act as anti-inflammatory agents, they have exciting potential value in treating diseases of inflammation like Alzheimer's, Parkinson's, and Huntington's diseases. Finally, I will discuss how all this affects you, the reader, as we consider what you can take by way of foods and supplements to optimize the remarkable potential for longevity and health discovered in resveratrol and other xeno factors. My discussion will include safety and quality control, as well as specific dosages. I also will include a unique formula for balancing your life as well as your diet.

It is ironic that humankind has been searching for and developing exotic ways to enhance longevity for millennia, when the longevity factor may literally have been under our noses all the time and activated in the very same plants with which we have coexisted and coevolved for millions of years. This is one of the most absorbing stories in contemporary biology and the latest chapter in that search, and in the exciting emerging research that may significantly contribute to a longer, stronger, and healthier human life span.

Part I

Discovery, Xenohormesis, and Xeno Factors

Chapter 1

The Origins of Life

In the beginning God created the heaven and the earth. And the earth was without form, and void. . . . And God said, Let the waters bring forth abundantly the moving creature that hath life . . . and every living creature that moveth . . . : and God saw that it was good.

—GENESIS, CHAPTER 1

On the last day of February 1953, students and faculty members from the Cavendish Laboratory at England's University of Cambridge were having lunch at the Eagle pub, drinking Green King beer and enjoying the bar, with its graffiti from World War II airmen. At the top of the lunch hour, Francis Crick, a thirty-seven-year-old physicist turned biologist who had not yet earned his PhD, bounded in and loudly announced to his colleague, the zoologist turned geneticist James Watson, "We have found the secret of life!" Indeed they had. That morning, the two young scientists had deciphered the structure of deoxyribonucleic acid (DNA)—two strands of sugar connected by paired molecules called bases—an accomplishment for which they would later win the Nobel Prize.

That structure, a "double helix" that can "unzip" to make copies of itself, was the finding that confirmed that DNA carried the hereditary code of life. Crick and Watson immediately published their findings in the scientific journal *Nature,* and capped a rather academic, dry account of DNA's structure with one of the most famous understatements in the history of science: "It has not escaped our notice that the specific pairings we have postulated immediately suggest a possible copying mechanism for genetic material"—that is, of life.

Fifty years later, in 2003, another landmark paper appeared in the same prestigious international journal, also from a Cambridge laboratory, but this time in Massachusetts. The head of the Paul F. Glenn Laboratories for the Biological Mechanisms of Aging at Harvard Medical School, David Sinclair, and his associates published a paper entitled "Small Molecule Activators of Sirtuins Extend *Saccharomyces cerevisiae* Lifespan." A year later, another peer-reviewed journal, *Molecular Microbiology,* published their follow-up article, "Small Molecules That Regulate Lifespan: Evidence for Xenohormesis."

Sinclair explained that certain plants can increase production of specialized molecules during times of stress, such as drought or increased ultraviolet radiation from the sun. When consumed by animals, these plant molecules, which Sinclair called xeno factors, were found to interact with the animals' genes and impart amazing health benefits. Most astonishing was the observation that these laboratory animals lived substantially longer—in some cases, up to 50 percent longer—than their average expected life span. Tests for cell damage indicated that they were also much healthier, with fewer occurrences of cancer, heart disease, and brain cell deterioration than is normally seen with aging (see figure 1).

This discovery, which has since been confirmed in laboratories at MIT and the University of California, San Francisco, is revolutionizing our ideas of how and why we age. Because human DNA has important basic similarities with animal DNA, we also possess similar genes that can be activated by eating these specialized plant molecules. For the first time in human history, there is real evidence that we can use this process to slow aging and live not only longer but healthier.

In the Beginning

When I considered that the same stressed plant molecules could prolong life in yeast (evolutionarily approximately one billion years old),

LIFE SPAN EXTENSION

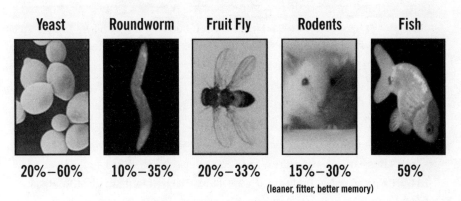

Yeast	Roundworm	Fruit Fly	Rodents	Fish
20%–60%	10%–35%	20%–33%	15%–30% (leaner, fitter, better memory)	59%

FIGURE 1 Extension of life span by xeno factors.

fish (500 million years old), and mammals (200 million years old), I became perplexed. What could possibly be the biological connection between the lowly yeast and humankind? To solve this scientific co-nundrum, I found myself going farther and farther back in time, asking more questions. What are the most basic molecular factors that all living things have in common? And is there a common biological language that makes all cells form, grow, function, reproduce, and die?

This incredible story of discovery may well begin with the formation of the universe nearly 14 billion years ago, when all the matter, energy, and space in what is now the observable universe were contained in a single infinitely dense point. From that point came a cataclysmic, fiery explosion commonly referred to as the "big bang" (see figure 2), in which space expanded and particles of the embryonic universe formed. These particles coalesced to form the billions of galaxies that now make up the universe, including our own Milky Way, with its own billions of stars.

After the big bang, incomprehensible amounts of heat and radiation were released and subatomic particles were formed—including protons, neutrons, electrons, quarks, and baryons—all of which would become the building blocks of life as we know it. This material cooled until approximately 4.5 billion years ago, when the earth was formed.

Timeline   **Present Day**

0	1 sec	3 min	300,000 yr	1 bil yr	15 bil yr
Expansion from the size of an atom to an explosion of superhot atomic particles, followed by rapid cooling.	Still very hot, now a "fog" of atomic particles.	Atomic particles come together to form atoms of the lightest elements, hydrogen and helium.	Gravity begins to push the lighter elements together to form clouds of gas, and pressure forms, making heavier elements and stars begin to form.	Galaxies of stars cluster and form new stars and planets.	

FIGURE 2 The big bang theory explains that a cosmic explosion at the beginning of time expanded space containing matter in all directions. As this matter cooled, gravity and pressure allowed atoms to form into elements and eventually into the planets and stars we see today.

Initially, as recorded in Genesis, water did completely cover the globe. There was no oxygen, only intense cosmic radiation, turbulent seas, volcanic eruptions, and frequent meteoric bombardments from outer space. During the next billion years, primary elements needed to support life were formed, including carbon, oxygen, nitrogen, phosphorus, sulfur, magnesium, calcium, copper, and iron.

The Origin of Life

It was indeed from the waters that life on our planet began. Charles Darwin, in 1871, made the suggestion that the original spark of life may have begun in a "warm little pond with all sorts of ammonia and phosphoric salts, light, heat, and electricity present, so that a protein compound was chemically formed that was ready to undergo still more complex changes." These changes led to a crucial step in the formation of life: the development of a more complex molecule that was itself capable of reproducing itself. The latest research now indicates that *ribonucleic acid,* or *RNA*—a molecule similar to DNA—may have been the first complex molecule on which life was developed. Like

DNA, RNA contains genetic information, but it also performs chemical reactions, like some proteins. But proteins cannot reproduce on their own; that was the amazing feat accomplished by RNA.

RNA is the common ancestor that has given rise to the major cell lines of life. The first of these belongs to a type of bacteria called prokaryotes, which lack a cellular nucleus. Bacteria that are two to three billion years old have been discovered in ancient rocks from Australia. They have survived throughout the millennia due to the simplicity of their design and their ability to become dormant for long periods at a time.

The second cell line is the eukaryote. These cells contain a cell nucleus, separated from the rest of the cell by a membrane; this nucleus is where the cell's DNA is housed. The word *eukaryote,* which derives from ancient Greek, refers to the "true nucleus." Eukaryotic cells are the basic building blocks of all animal life, from single-celled organisms like amoebas to complex human beings. Interestingly, fungi, mushrooms, and yeast also have eukaryote cell types; this is why the study of yeast cells has been found helpful in understanding many human cellular functions.

Cells of the third type, the archaebacteria, a subset of prokaryotes, have been referred to as "life's extremists." These cells inhabit some of the most forbidding and remote environments on the planet, including the depths of hot springs, or extremely alkaline or acidic waters. They live in the mud of marshes and at the very bottom of the ocean, and they thrive in places hostile to all other life-forms.

The first animal cells appeared about 1.5 billion years ago, single-cell organisms that were able to reproduce. Protected by a cell membrane formed of protein and fats, they were also able to use raw materials that could be converted into energy, and to respond to changes in environmental temperature, acidity, or nutrient levels. These reactions were facilitated by specialized reactive molecules called *enzymes.*

Enzymes, which we will learn more about, are specialized proteins that act as catalysts and can help alter and form other more complex proteins and nucleic acids that make up RNA and DNA. They are critical to the function and survival of all living things. In his research, David Sinclair discovered one specific enzyme critical to longevity.

With the formation of algae and multicellular structures like jellyfish and plankton, the stage was set for the evolution of higher organisms. Yeast was formed approximately 900 million years ago. Although for thousands of years it was used for fermenting alcohol and making bread, yeast wasn't known to be a living organism until Louis Pasteur confirmed it in the 1860s. Yeast subsequently played a critical role, as we shall see, in the study of aging. Six hundred million years ago, the first animals, invertebrates such as sponges, jellyfish, worms, and insects, made their appearance on our planet. Plants eventually evolved from ancient green algae and populated the earth approximately 400 million years ago, shortly before the appearance of vertebrate animals about 380 million years ago (see figure 3).

After the abrupt eradication of the dinosaurs about 65 million years ago, following a dramatic drop in the earth's temperature, mammals began to proliferate, leading to the appearance of our humanlike ancestors approximately 2 million to 3 million years ago. Modern humankind is but a flash in the evolutionary night, being approximately 400,000 years old, with a recorded history less than 15,000 years old. Carl Sagan put this in perspective when he speculated on the evolution of human intelligence in his book *The Dragons of Eden*. He constructed a timeline in which the period from the big bang to the present moment was represented by a 365-day calendar year. In that scenario, all of recorded human history occupies the last ten seconds of December 31; the time from the waning of the Middle Ages to the present would occupy little more than one second.

Although our time on earth as a species is so short, there is a corollary to this. Since all the constituents that would eventually come together for our embodiment were present in the big bang, we really trace our lineage to a moment 13.7 billion to 15 billion years ago. Since all matter derives from that initial burst, each of us is formed of the same primordial dust that subsequently became stars; every living thing carries within it elements that evolved and reconstituted until they finally formed what we are today.

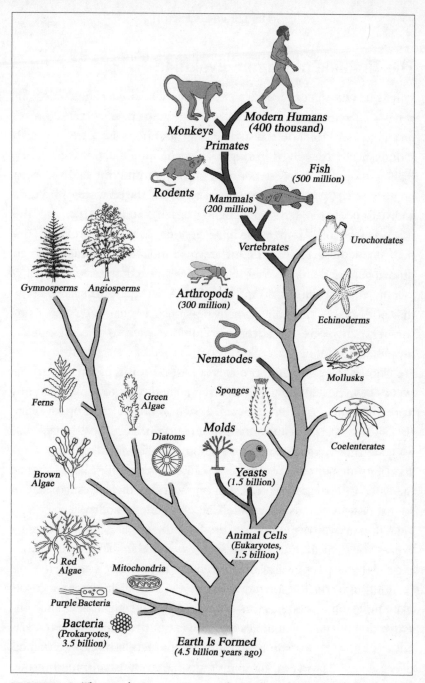

FIGURE 3 The evolutionary tree and timeline from the formation of earth to modern man showing the common genetic linkage of yeast, worms, fish, mice, and humans.

The Timeline of Human Evolution

Why is this lineage so crucial to our story of how we can activate our genes to live longer and healthier by ingesting specific stressed plant products? Because it demonstrates how the various life-forms on earth synergistically coevolved throughout earth's multibillion-year history, making them intimately dependent on one another for survival. Most important, the genetic code that provides for the survival of bacteria and yeast is written in the same biological language that articulates the biochemistry of a human being. Scientific studies, therefore, conducted on these early forms of life may indeed be extrapolated to human beings, thanks to our shared DNA. Through the science of phylogeny, which studies relationships of DNA between species, we know that both plants and animals activate similar genetic mechanisms to survive in response to adverse conditions such as excessive heat, drought, and famine.

The concept of xenohormesis is based on the premise that our bodies have developed the ability to read and react to molecular cues from the plant world during times of environmental stress or adversity. By ingesting certain nutrients from environmentally stressed plants, we genetically activate our body's defenses to survive. This survival response results in cellular changes in our body controlled by genes and mediated by enzymes that can shift our everyday metabolism of sugars so that now we can use our stored fats as an energy source.

The survival response triggered by these plant molecules also causes the activation of animal *mitochondria,* the structures within the cell that act as powerhouses, or energy producers, allowing the mitochondria to release a larger amount of energy. Ultimately, stressed plant molecules—xeno factors—can stimulate health and enhance immune defenses in the animals that consume them, increasing the viability of those animals in a stressful environment. This strengthening effect is what David Sinclair and others have now confirmed both by documenting less disease and increased longevity in laboratory animals, and by isolating the genetic mechanisms at work.

This discovery is the by-product of yet another new scientific field heralded by Watson and Crick, molecular biology, which attempts to unravel the biochemistry of life's beginnings and the vast molecular web of interaction between plants and animals. In the last fifty years, more has been discovered about the secrets of both plant life and animal life than in the previous 15,000 years of recorded history. Since the early 1990s, researchers at the forefront of molecular biology have taken a Neil Armstrong–like "giant leap for mankind" toward finally unraveling the secrets of life—and how to prolong it.

Chapter 2

Molecular Pioneers and the Discovery of Longevity Genes

If I have seen farther, it is by standing on the shoulders of giants.

— ISAAC NEWTON, LETTER TO ROBERT HOOKE,
FEBRUARY 5, 1675

History is replete with examples of medical pioneers whose innovations and foresight were trivialized, ignored, challenged, or violently opposed by the establishment only to ultimately become accepted by society at large.

— DR. RONALD KLATZ, FOUNDER, THE AMERICAN
ACADEMY OF ANTI-AGING MEDICINE, 2008

In 1953, the same year that Watson and Crick launched the modern era of molecular biology, a former beekeeper from New Zealand, Edmund Hillary, scaled the previously insurmountable heights of Mount Everest. Both feats captured international attention and established new standards of accomplishment: the personal qualities of focus, intensity, perseverance against all odds and obstacles, ambition, and a burning competitiveness. And both triumphs drew on the failures and successes of those who had gone before. The discovery of xenohormesis is similarly predicated on the work of a long line of innovators.

Because the mechanisms by which xenohormetic plant molecules improve health and longevity in animals involve genes and their products, we must first understand something about DNA and the genes it comprises. Our story of molecular biology begins in 1859 with Charles Darwin and his now famous publication of *On the Origin of Species by Means of Natural Selection*. Upon returning from a two-year scientific expedition to the Galápagos Islands, Darwin used changes in the development of the beak of the finch to argue that all present-day creatures had indeed evolved into their present forms, and he provided the first plausible explanation of the means by which they did so: natural selection, or evolution. What is relevant for us here is that natural selection and the development of survival mechanisms were due to adaptation to stress.

Darwin recognized that in a world of limited resources, life consists of a fierce competition for survival, or, in his words, "a struggle for life." He also recognized that some species were "fitter," or better adapted to succeed in the prevailing environmental conditions, and this recognition led him to theorize that populations evolve over the course of generations through a process of natural selection. With the establishment of these basic concepts, the evolutionary ascent of *Homo sapiens* became based in science. Darwin himself knew full well that his idea of evolution driven by natural selection was incomplete. He recognized that offspring could differ in major ways from both parents and from their siblings. But he didn't know how those differences occurred or how they were transmitted over generations.

If Darwin had been aware of the work of the Austrian monk Gregor Mendel, he might have known that this problem had been solved three years earlier, in 1856. During frequent walks through the monastery garden in what is now the Czech Republic, Mendel had observed the simple traits of common pea plants growing in the garden. He noted that the flowers of these plants were either purple or white and the pods were either yellow or green—nothing in between. The stem of the plant was either long or short, and the seeds were either round or wrinkled. Altogether he observed seven different traits that never seemed to blend. His curiosity piqued, he put his mathematics and physics background to work crossbreeding and analyzing more than 28,000 different pea plants, their combinations, and their characteristics.

Mendel bred peas with green pods to peas with yellow pods and noted that their offspring all turned out to have green pods. However, when he bred this second generation with itself, 25 percent of the next generation turned out to have yellow pods. The same observation held true for height. After he bred long-stem peas with short-stem peas, the next generation was all tall, but 25 percent of the generation after that were short. His simple but elegant experiments in the monastery garden provided the framework for the subsequent field of genetics, the study of "the code of life." His basic observations formed the foundation for understanding why certain traits appear to skip generations, as observed by Darwin in the finches in the Galápagos Islands (see figure 4).

Modern evolutionary biology and the basis for molecular biology are predicated on three of Mendel's observations. First, each feature is

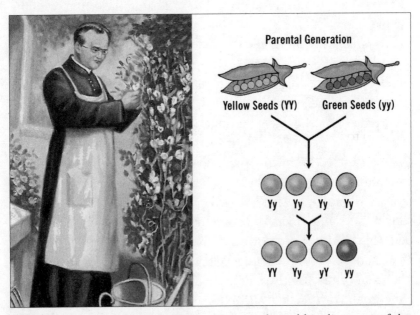

FIGURE 4 Gregor Mendel, the Austrian monk, and his discovery of the method of transmission of the genetic code in pea plants.

determined by some discrete "factor," which would later be called a gene, which passes on the information of heredity. Second, each gene within a species can exist in more than one version, called an allele. For example, the gene for seed shape in pea plants comes in two variations: one allele for a round seed shape and the other for a wrinkled seed shape. Third, Mendel perceived that in mixed pairs, one allele was dominant over the other. (In the case of seed shapes, round is dominant, and wrinkled is recessive.) These three principles summarize the essence of the method of transmission of the genetic code that contains, in chemical language, the recipe for all the traits we inherit at birth.

Another building block of molecular biology was set in place serendipitously in 1902, when a medical student at Columbia University named Walter Sutton discovered paired "blobs" within the nucleus of the cell. Using a new, more powerful microscope, he isolated these blobs, which turned out to be *chromosomes*. Chromosomes are the structures formed by coiled strands of DNA within the nucleus. They are arranged in pairs—twenty-three in humans. In most plant and animal cells, a different parent provides each half of the pair. Thus the idea of mixing different traits from different parents dovetailed with Mendel's ideas on pairing and mixing traits on a genetic level.

Approximately twenty years after Mendel's experiments with pea plants, Wilhelm Johannsen, a professor of botany at Copenhagen Agricultural College, assigned the word *gene* (meaning "origin" or "to give birth to") to the fundamental physical and functional unit that controls heredity. In addition, he referred to the particular set of genes possessed by an individual as its *genotype*. He also coined the term *phenotype:* an organism's actual physical characteristics such as height, weight, and hair color. The phenotype is to some degree molded by the environment. Identical twins have the same genotype, since their genes are identical, but they never have the same phenotype, due to the strong influence of environmental factors such as infection, trauma, and stress. These concepts elaborated by Johannsen were fundamental to understanding the theory of evolution postulated by Darwin.

The next major advance in our story of genetics occurred in New York City. In the 1920s, a biology student at Columbia College, who would later win a Nobel Prize, began working with the *Drosophila,* or fruit fly. Just as Mendel and Johannsen had observed different characteristics when breeding peas and beans, Hermann Muller now observed significant anatomical changes in fruit flies after blasting them with ionizing radiation. He noticed that some now had long wings or short wings, and some were now missing body parts. There was also a new difference in the male-to-female ratio. As a result of his observations, Muller began publicizing the likely dangers of radiation exposure in humans, particularly for physicians and technicians who operated X-ray equipment. In 1946 he won the Nobel Prize for the discovery that X-rays can induce genetic mutations. This is important because xeno factors also have the ability to influence and in some cases repair damaged DNA within cells, thereby reversing or blocking genetic mutations that can occur with disease such as cancer.

Curiously, the next segment of important research on our way to the xeno factor involves bread mold. George Wells Beadle, from Wahoo, Nebraska, joined the "fly" lab at the California Institute of Technology to follow up on Muller's work on fruit fly genetics. Beadle collaborated with a chemist, Edward Tatum, from the University of Chicago, to study the genetics of the fungus, an organism more than a billion years old, using Muller's technique of ionizing radiation. By exposing bread mold fungus to X-rays, they caused mutations in the fungus just as Muller had with his fruit flies. In a series of experiments, Beadle and Tatum showed that these mutations cause changes in specific enzymes. These findings led the two researchers to propose a direct link between genes and enzymes. This became known as the "one gene, one enzyme" hypothesis: the idea that a specific section of genetic code is responsible for making one and only one type of enzyme, which carries out a specific biochemical function. For this research, Beadle and Tatum shared a 1958 Nobel Prize. The discovery of the relationship between enzymes—the protein catalysts responsible for all chemical reactions essential for life—and the genes that make them was another fundamental building block in the discovery of xeno factors.

A crucial next step was taken by the brilliant Austrian physicist Irwin Schrödinger, who won the Nobel Prize in Physics in 1933. In considering the great unsolved problems in science, he published a well-known book in 1944 entitled *What Is Life?* In it he wrote: "It is these chromosomes, DNA strands formed into paired genes found in the nucleus of cells, that contain in some kind of code the script for the entire pattern of the individual's future development and of its functioning in the mature state." This concept of paired genes encoded with a particular biochemical pattern was crucial for future observations, as we will see.

Another piece of the puzzle was added in 1944 by Oswald Avery, a Canadian physician and biochemist, who showed that a harmless form of bacteria could be changed to a killer by adding DNA from a culture of virulent bacteria. Furthermore, he recognized that DNA was the active substance that determined the specific characteristics of the cell. DNA molecules are formed by various combinations of only four different building blocks called *nucleotides*—adenine (A), guanine (G), thymine (T), and cytosine (C)—although a list of the various combinations of these units would fill two hundred telephone books!

Erwin Chargaff provided the next scientific piece of the puzzle. In 1951 he observed that "the amount of nucleotide adenine equals that of thymine, and the amount of guanine equals that of cytosine." This observation, unappreciated at the time, was critical to the subsequent understanding of the configuration of the double helix. These nucleotide building blocks are cross-linked like the rungs of a ladder, and these links can be easily broken during cell division, allowing the two strands of the DNA molecule to separate and act as a template to form exact copies of themselves. Thus genetic information coded in the DNA can be used by the cell for reproduction and for the formation of the protein building blocks of all living structures (see figure 5).

By assimilating all of these discoveries, and by incorporating the X-ray images of DNA produced by Rosalind Franklin, who worked in a competing lab and nearly discovered the double helix herself, Watson and Crick conceived their astonishing and elegant solution to the mys-

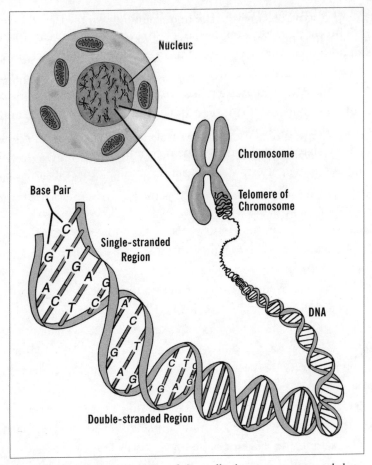

FIGURE 5 This illustration of the cell, chromosomes, and double helix DNA structure with the base pair nucleotide connections shows that the adenine and thymine pair, and the guanine and cytosine pair, are always matched throughout the structure.

tery of life on that frigid day in February 1953. Using bits of paper and metal attached to different-sized rods, they found that the pieces of the jigsaw puzzle finally fit. The secret of the double helix of DNA coiled inside each chromosome was unraveled, and by standing on the shoulders of the scientific giants who had preceded them, Watson and Crick launched the modern era of molecular biology.

These discoveries provide the underpinnings for the equally exciting inquiry into how and why we age—and what we can do about it. The fact is that DNA and the genes it forms are the storehouse for more than one billion years of organisms learning how to adapt and survive in an ever-changing environment. The complete story of the secrets they hold about longevity has yet to be written, but exciting discoveries have already led to new ways of looking at cancer, heart disease, and Alzheimer's disease, and what we can do proactively to prevent them. The emerging benefits will change the way we live, work, and plan for retirement, as well as the shape of tomorrow's society and the very future of our species.

Chapter 3

Causes of Aging

The belief that aging is still an unsolved problem in biology is no longer true.

—MICROBIOLOGIST LEONARD HAYFLICK, 2007

Why do we age? Why do all living creatures have a finite period of existence? What is the nature of the clock of life whose alarm we can't turn off? As a species, human beings have now survived for 400,000 years, but not as individuals. Still, we can consider ourselves fortunate compared with some life-forms that measure their life spans in mere days. Among animals, the gastrotrich, a minute sea creature, has the briefest life expectancy—about three days—whereas the giant tortoise can live more than 170 years. Plants can live for extraordinary periods, like the Methuselah tree, a bristlecone pine found in California, which is estimated to be 4,725 years old. People fall somewhere in the middle range. In the Bible, we are told that Moses lived to 120 years. Jeanne Calment, however, outlived Moses by two years; born in Arles, France, in 1875, she died in 1997 at the age of 122. Her secret? She recommended walking and two glasses of red wine each day.

Still, the average life expectancy of an American born today is only 77.9 years. That's respectable, but it's not as long as the life expectancy of citizens born in forty-one other countries. The pocket-sized country of Andorra, located between France and Spain, tops the list at 83.5 years. As we will see, the natural upper limit of the life span may be significantly higher, based on tests with laboratory animals and an analysis of people who lived beyond 100. In fact, many scientists in antiaging research believe it may be possible to consistently prolong life to the age of Moses and Jeanne Calment as science advances over the next twenty to thirty years.

Lest you think this is science fiction, we have already seen an increase in life span of about three months every year since the mid-nineteenth century. This is generally attributed to the industrialization of food production, which created a readily available food supply, and to the introduction of childhood immunizations and antibiotics. But some researchers believe that even with the most advanced medical care, the average human life span has very little room to increase further. In fact, there is evidence that in some countries, like Russia, life span can even backslide. The discovery of substances that could extend life is therefore both very intriguing and very controversial, and must be examined in the context of scientific trial and error and, most important, through confirmation by other scientists, the litmus test of scientific progress.

What Is Normal Aging?

Hall of Famer Leroy "Satchel" Paige, who was still pitching in major-league baseball in his fifties, once asked, "How old would you be if you didn't know how old you were?" Having myself competed in Ironman Triathlon events at ages sixty and sixty-eight, I have seen firsthand what gerontologists have long known: chronological age—the number of years you've lived—doesn't necessarily correlate with physiological age. If we can prevent chronic diseases and disability through diet, exercise, and avoiding environmental hazards such as pollution and pesticides, we can stay much younger than our chronological age. Of course, coming from a family blessed with long life in its genetic history can also help.

Professional wrestler Bruno Sammartino, a patient and friend of mine, is the best example I know of someone who remains almost as youthful as when he began his career more than fifty years ago. Considered by many to be the greatest wrestler of all time, "the Italian Superman" overcame such daunting threats as Hulk Hogan, Killer Kowalski, Gorilla Monsoon, and countless others during his seven-year run as world champion. Bruno sold out New York City's Madison Square Garden a record 187 times.

After concluding his career with an induction into the Professional Wrestling Hall of Fame, Bruno has maintained an exercise regimen matching that of the famous fitness expert Jack LaLanne. Weight and aerobic training remain a part of his everyday life, as do a deep devotion to his faith and his wife. Over the years Bruno gravitated to a diet high in xeno factors, consuming two glasses of red wine every night with his dinner and regularly eating fresh fruit, vegetables, and fish. He also has maintained an ideal weight and never smoked. At age seventy-three, his youthful physique, mental acuity, and physical prowess remain remarkably intact (see figure 6). As we will discuss in chapter 20, he has managed to attain balance in his life and his diet, making his golden years truly golden.

Certainly aging does not manifest itself in the same way in every person. Genetic predisposition and lifestyle are major additional influences on aging. To discover just what happens to various organs as people age, the National Institute on Aging supported the Baltimore

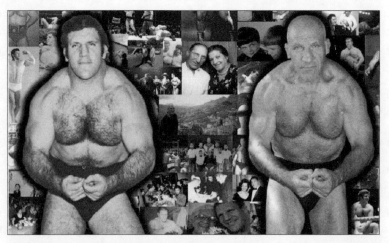

FIGURE 6 Professional wrestler Bruno Sammartino at age twenty-seven (left) and at age seventy (right).

Longitudinal Study of Aging, which has tracked more than 1,400 men and women, ranging in age from their twenties to their nineties.

Although the study shows a wide variety in rates of decline, the following generalities can be made:

TABLE 1 How Different Organs Are Affected by Aging

Heart	The heart wall thickens, gradually losing its effectiveness as a pump. Maximum oxygen consumption during exercise declines with each decade of adult life by about 10 percent in men and 7.5 percent in women.
Arteries	Cholesterol and calcium build up, thickening and stiffening the arteries. The decrease in elasticity and the narrowing of the arteries lead to high blood pressure.
Lungs	Between the ages of twenty and seventy, maximum breathing capacity declines by approximately 40 percent.
Brain	A gradual decrease in the number of brain cells leads to selective impairment, particularly in memory.
Bladder	The bladder gradually loses its tone, and incontinence or loss of control of urine may occur as the tissues weaken, particularly in women.
Body fat	Body fat gradually increases until middle age. It then usually stabilizes until late life, when body weight tends to decline. Elderly individuals lose not only body fat but also muscle and thus develop sagging skin.
Muscles	Between the ages of thirty and seventy, muscle mass declines by approximately 22 percent for women and 23 percent for men. (Exercise slows, and even reverses, this rate of loss.)
Bones	Bone density and minerals are lost, particularly in women at menopause. This loss accelerates and leads to osteoporosis and fractures.
Sight and hearing	Both begin to fade in the forties. There is increased susceptibility to glare and greater difficulty in seeing at low illumination. In older people, high-frequency tones are lost so that impairment with background noise becomes substantial. Hearing declines more quickly in men than in women.

All of these abnormalities occur eventually, but they can be greatly delayed and at times prevented by appropriate diet and exercise.

Theories of Aging

Many theories have been proposed to explain why we age and eventually die; however, none has gained supremacy. In fact, Caleb Finch, PhD, who studies the causes of aging at the University of Southern California, has noted, "Next to the miracle of life itself, aging and death are perhaps the greatest mysteries." Nevertheless, theories of aging can be divided into two groups: error theories and programmed theories.

Error Theories of Aging

Perhaps the most notable error theory concerns *free radicals.* In every cell, there are hundreds of mitochondria, tiny organelles that convert oxygen and glucose into adenosine triphosphate (ATP). ATP is the energy-releasing molecule needed for almost all cellular reactions. In the normal process of "burning" oxygen and carbohydrates, mitochondria form by-products called free radicals, created when the mitochondria combine oxygen with hydrogen to form water and an oxygen molecule escapes with an extra electron.

These oxygen atoms with a free or unpaired electron (free "radicals") are unstable and break down into several additional types of free radicals that attempt to "steal" electrons from other molecules. Sometimes this is helpful, as when free radicals destroy bacteria or other invaders. However, in excess, free radicals can damage the membranes of cells, the proteins within cells, and even the DNA itself (see figure 7). There are other sources of free radicals besides the mitochondria, however, such as sun exposure, radiation, tobacco smoke, and other environmental factors. In fact, radiation therapy to treat cancer depends on free radicals generated by the radiation to kill the cancer cells. Free radicals have been implicated in all aspects of aging, from degenerative disorders to cancer, cataracts, atherosclerosis, and brain degeneration, as we will see.

To neutralize these free radicals that cause damage through *oxida-*

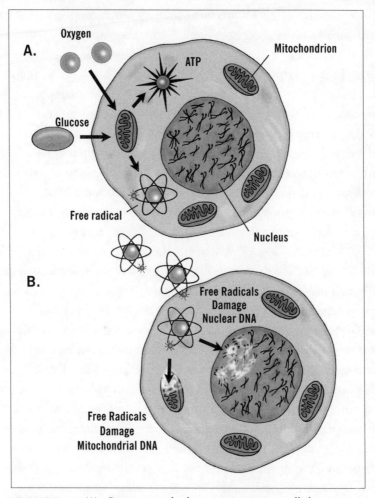

FIGURE 7 (A) Oxygen and glucose generate cellular energy (ATP) and in the process form destructive free radicals. (B) Excessive free radicals damage cellular membranes, mitochondria, and DNA.

tion, cells call upon *antioxidants.* In a healthy body, nutrients like vitamins C and E, along with various enzymes, are powerful antioxidants that normally prevent damage by the free radicals. Antioxidants are now often added to food and drinks, which are then called "functional foods." Marketed as containing nutrients to protect cells from damage due to oxidation, 1,013 products making "high antioxidant" claims were introduced in 2006. The Mars chocolate company recently put an antioxidant label on its Dove chocolate and saw its business double in a year. In the first three months of 2007, more products with antioxidant claims came out than in all of 2004. The best source of antioxidants, however, isn't packaged foods, according to nutritionists, but natural (and preferably organically) grown fruits and vegetables.

Another error theory of aging is that of cross-linking. People who have elevated blood sugar, particularly diabetics, are subject to developing what are called advanced glycation end products (AGEs). In this process, glucose molecules attach themselves to proteins or fats. Anyone who has basted a Thanksgiving turkey and watched the skin turn brown and stiff is seeing AGEs in action. The cross-linked glucose-protein material is responsible for the stiffening and has a similar effect on human skin and on the connective tissue that supports our joints, tendons, and internal organs. The number of AGEs increases with age and accelerates the process of aging and organ failure. This is especially evident in diabetics who develop premature heart, kidney, and/or blood vessel damage, plus cataracts—all accelerated by AGEs.

A third error theory is that of repetitive damage to the DNA in the nucleus and the mitochondria of the cell. Each of the trillions of cells in the body strives to maintain a balance between a continual assault by oxygen-free radicals, the sun's ultraviolet radiation, and other toxic agents, and the normal mechanisms needed to repair the damaged DNA. When the repair system is overwhelmed, genetic mutations in the cell's DNA accumulate over time. This results in cellular deterioration, malfunction, and even cancer. Damage to the mitochondrial DNA is thought to cause many muscle disorders, as well as inflammatory diseases such as Alzheimer's.

Error theories include the belief that over time, cells simply begin to function poorly and wear out. Dr. Henry Lodge, coauthor of *Younger Next Year,* notes that "most aging is just the 'dry rot' we program into our cells by sedentary living, junk food, and stress." He makes the interesting observation that although the body is composed of trillions of cells, most live only a few weeks or months, then die and are replaced in an endless cycle. Although this isn't entirely true for all organs (such as the brain and heart), our cells do create a "new" body approximately every three months—leaving many opportunities for errors in cell reproduction. Cancer is an example of just such a mistake.

Programmed Theories of Aging

These theories involve loss of organ function at a specific rate as we age. One such theory of aging involves the endocrine glands, which produce hormones such as estrogen, testosterone, growth and thyroid hormones, DHEA, and melatonin. All of these hormones gradually decrease with age.

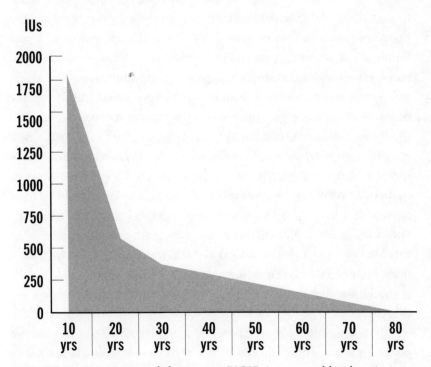

FIGURE 8 Human growth hormone (HGH) is secreted by the pituitary gland. HGH levels peak during adolescence and subsequently decrease with age. The levels of HGH after age thirty decline approximately 15 percent per decade.

For example, human growth hormone from the pituitary gland normally peaks at around age thirty and then gradually declines thereafter (figure 8). A study by David Rudman in the *New England Journal of Medicine* in 1990 showed that in elderly patients, growth hormone supplements led to improved memory, decreased age-related stomach fat, thicker muscles and skin, and an overall feeling of wellness. In a follow-up article in 2003, also in the *New England Journal of Medicine,* Mary Lee Vance expressed concerns about Rudman's study because of the lack of evaluation of long-term side effects and also the fact that more recent similar studies had shown no strength improvement. Although still controversial, today human growth hormone supplementation has become an underground cult movement.

Hormones, produced by various glands, are chemicals that control the activities of organs and other parts of the body. For example, the male sex hormone, testosterone, formed in the testicles, has a profound effect on muscle size and strength, as well as sex drive and mood. Testosterone production peaks in early adulthood, then tapers off as we age. The National Institute on Aging is investigating the role of testosterone supplementation in delaying or preventing frailty in the elderly. Similarly, the female sex hormone, estrogen, made in a woman's ovaries, has a powerful effect on bone growth and development; it also regulates the menstrual cycle. Deficiencies in this hormone may result in osteoporosis and menopausal symptoms. Other hormones such as DHEA and melatonin are also touted as antiaging, and at times even miraculous in their effects on general health. All of these hormones can be measured in the blood. If they are low, replacement can indeed be life transforming.

A decline in immunity also falls under programmed aging. The immune system, composed of the tonsils and adenoids, thymus gland, lymph nodes, spleen, lymphatic vessels, and cells in the bone marrow, produces powerful blood cells and substances that neutralize or kill invaders such as bacteria, viruses, and other foreign bodies. When our immune system is strong, we have few colds or infections and our energy level is high. When we are exposed to the high bacterial count in a crowded airplane, for example, we become sick to varying degrees, depending on the strength of our immune system. With age, the organs in the immune system gradually fail, so that we become much more susceptible. Fortunately, there are ways to enhance the immune system to better fight infections, such as including natural xeno factors in our foods.

Mental stress and depression have long been known to weaken the immune system. In ancient Rome, Galen, the physician to the gladiators, observed that bereavement and depression from the death of a spouse could itself lead to an early death. Beginning in the 1980s, a new field called psychoneuroimmunology emerged to decipher the biochemical connections between the mind and body. The biblical statement "As a man thinketh, so he shall be" may well be accurate. It turns out that when we are depressed, our thoughts and feelings suppress cells in our immune system, increasing our susceptibility to sickness. When we use positive thinking, meditation, and prayer and have a strong family support system, we are much more effective at warding off disease.

The final programmed theory of aging relates to telomeres—repetitive DNA sequences at the end of chromosomes. Like the plastic covering on the ends of shoelaces, these telomeres help to keep the chromosome intact. Each time cells divide, our telomeres get shorter. It is thought that over time the telomeres become so short that their function is disrupted, leading to cells that no longer divide and proliferate. By measuring the length of telomeres, we can get some idea of how many cell divisions have already occurred and how many remain before a particular cell can no longer replicate.

This biological clock keeps track of the cell's age and serves as a molecular marker to measure cellular division. As the telomeres fray, cells wear out, and the organism dies. This raises two important questions: How do the cells that make up the next generation—the male sperm and the female egg—avoid this fate, and how do cancer cells continue to grow?

Drs. Jerry Shay and Woody Wright, professors in the department of cell biology at the University of Texas Southwestern Medical Center, have provided the answer. They discovered that an enzyme called telomerase enables cells to replace the lost telomeres and then to divide indefinitely. In the case of the reproductive cells and stem cells (the master cells, with the ability to grow into any one of the body's more than two hundred cell types), this is a necessary and important process, but when the telomerase gene is activated erroneously in other cells, it can allow tumors to grow unchecked. Cancer research has been focusing on drugs to block telomerase, and the precise role of telomere shortening in aging and cancer is one of several research avenues that scientists continue to pursue vigorously.

In reviewing these various theories of aging, it becomes immediately apparent that aging has multiple causes. In mammals, aging is dependent in large part on the type of maintenance mechanisms evoked to slow this decay and deterioration of our cells and organs. I'm referring to the repair of DNA, defense systems against oxygen free radicals, enhancement of the immune response, removal of defective proteins and mutated cells, and the detoxification of harmful chemicals in our diet.

These maintenance mechanisms bring us directly back to the xeno factor, for researchers are finding that the plant chemicals found in xeno factors perform *all* of these functions. By activating specific mechanisms within our cells, they help to control inflammation, regulate cell survival, repair cells, and prevent cell death. As antioxidants, they work to enhance the all-important performance of the immune and endocrine systems.

Chapter 4

Calorie Restriction and Longevity

To lengthen thy life, lessen thy meals.

—BENJAMIN FRANKLIN

Experiments in our laboratory and several others have shown that the life span of an animal can be stretched by means of special diets.

—CLIVE MCCAY, 1935

Clive M. McCay, a nutritional scientist at Cornell University in New York, was one of the first and most successful scientific investigators in the antiaging field. In the 1930s, he sought to determine if calorie restriction would extend the life span by posing himself a question: if we slow the growth and development of an animal, do we also slow its decline? McCay conducted the first widely recognized scientific study to demonstrate that a calorie-restricted diet (but not a diet reduced in nutrients) did enable animals to live longer. He fed a group of rats a diet containing 20 percent indigestible cellulose, which reduced their caloric intake by approximately 40 percent, and found that it extended their life span by as much as 40 percent to 50 percent. Not only did the diet dramatically slow the rate of aging, but it also delayed the onset of diseases related to aging such as cancer, heart disease, and brain disease.

McCay's longest-lived calorie-restricted rats survived for forty-eight months, while his "control" (by including the control, or placebo, arm of the study, more reliable data are obtained) animals, who were fed a normal diet, died at the expected age of thirty months. Later experiments by other researchers kept rats alive for more than fifty-nine months—almost twice the normal life span. Since the 1930s, scientists around the world have confirmed the powerful effects of calorie restriction on animals. The same result has been observed in almost every laboratory animal tested. Yeast, worms, flies, mice, rats, and fish—all have responded to calorie restriction by living longer, with a lower incidence of most age-associated diseases. This approach has consistently proven to be the most effective way of extending the maximum life span of animals. It has also been discovered that the effects of calorie restriction are dose dependent—that is, the greater the degree of calorie restriction, the greater its effects, provided that the animal consumes balanced nutrients and eats enough to avoid starvation.

As one might imagine, this information has sparked the efforts of scientist hoping to replicate the animal test results in humans. The major problem is that a person needs to overcome a lifetime of eating habits (as well as hunger pangs) to obtain these potential benefits. The Calorie Restriction Society, a nonprofit organization that advocates this diet and lifestyle, estimates that a person needs to maintain a body weight of approximately 25 percent less than the medically established ideal weight. In terms of calorie consumption, this means approximately 40 percent less per day than the normal recommended diet. For women, dietitians and nutritionists usually recommend around 2,000 calories per day, and for men, 2,500 calories. This is quite variable, depending on body mass and activity level.

The risks and discomforts of such a diet, especially if it is not balanced, are many—including unattractive appearance changes, diminished bone mass, cold sensitivity, reduced energy reserves, and constant hunger. Severe calorie restriction also can cause menstrual irregularity and interfere with reproductive function in women, as well as reduce muscle mass, decrease testosterone in men, and slow wound healing. If one chooses to participate in such a diet, it must be nutritionally balanced in terms of carbohydrates, fats, and proteins. Needless to say, if you opt for such a restricted diet, you may live longer, but your quality of life may also be greatly diminished.

Human Evidence for the Benefits of Calorie Restriction

Nearly two hundred years before McCay conducted his experiments, Benjamin Franklin observed, "To lengthen thy life, lessen thy meals." With two-thirds of the American population currently either overweight or obese, his words ring powerfully today. So what does the evidence show in people?

Because of the suffering associated with severe calorie restriction, it has been difficult to design human experiments in this area. Still, several studies have been conducted that are worth noting. Physiologist Ancel Keys carried out one of the earliest at the University of Minnesota in the 1950s. He compared sixty volunteers who ate an average daily diet of 1,500 calories for three years with a control group who consumed 2,300 calories per day. Although the study was inconclusive as concerns longevity, it did demonstrate that the calorie-restricted group was healthier. (Keys, incidentally, lived to be one hundred.) Its members made fewer visits to the infirmary, for example, and blood tests also showed them to be healthier than the control group.

Another experiment performed an unintended evaluation of human calorie restriction. In 1991 four women and four men were sealed inside an enclosed artificial environment called Biosphere 2, covering more than three acres near Tucson, Arizona. The experiment was intended to see if a self-sustaining environment could be built to support the lives of eight people and the various plants and animals placed in it. This could provide interesting information about the possibility of living in such an environment in outer space, for example. The eight crew members were all experts in diverse areas, including botany, zoology, farming, and human health, and all were in excellent physical shape. The experiment, which was planned to last for two years, soon captured the world's attention because of an unforeseen problem with the design. Before long, it became clear that the amount of plant life in the biosphere could not produce the oxygen needed for the crew. In addition, the amount of food produced would result in severe calorie restriction. In the end, a decision was made to replenish the oxygen, but not the food.

One member of the crew, Dr. Roy Walford, was a pioneer in antiaging research and very familiar with the work of Clive McCay at Cornell. Walford persuaded the other members to do their own calorie-restricted experiment. The crew consumed a low-calorie diet of vegetables, fruits, nuts, grains, and beans, with small amounts of meat, dairy, and eggs. They experienced an average weight loss of 18 percent and decreased their body mass 19 percent for the men and 13 percent for the women. Additionally, their blood pressure went down about 25 percent on average, and blood sugar values and cholesterol were also lowered significantly. These numbers all resembled those of animals that had been placed on a similar calorie-restricted diet. Despite the severe conditions and weight loss, all the crew members of Biosphere 2 remained very healthy and were able to sustain a normal level of physical and mental activity throughout the entire two years of confinement.

Another well-documented study of calorie restriction evaluated dietary habits in a part of Japan known for its inhabitants' longevity. Researchers found that both children and adults in Okinawa consumed between 20 percent and 30 percent fewer calories than the national average. Okinawan death rates from stroke, cancer, and heart disease were lower by approximately 60 percent, and the number of centenarians on the island was forty times greater than that of the northeast part of Japan, where calorie intake was normal. Again, these results are consistent with animal studies showing that calorie restriction increases the life span and reduces the incidence and severity of age-related diseases.

In 2006, in the *Journal of the American Medical Association (JAMA),* Dr. Leonie Heilbronn and her associates reported the effect of six months of calorie restriction in forty-eight men. In this study, patients were randomly divided into two groups. Heilbronn restricted calories by 25 percent in one group and 12.5 percent in the other, whose members increased their exercise. She found significantly reduced blood sugar and insulin levels, and lower body temperature, in both groups compared with controls that were not calorie restricted.

Heilbronn also found that in those whose diets were restricted, cellular DNA appeared to be healthier, with fewer areas of damage.

In August 2007 three studies seemed to confirm that calorie restriction in humans, as in animals, adds to longevity. The first appeared in the *American Journal of Cardiology*. Scientists looked at the heart function of twenty-five people who had been calorie restricted for about six years. They ate 1,400 to 2,000 nutritionally balanced calories per day and were compared with a matched control group that ate a typical 2,000 to 3,000 calories daily. Using ultrasonic imaging to evaluate heart function, scientists found that the calorie-restricted hearts were more elastic and resembled hearts fifteen years younger than their actual age.

Two additional studies published simultaneously in the *New England Journal of Medicine* were even more convincing. Investigators from the University of Utah and Göteborg University in Sweden studied a total of twenty thousand obese people over a period of seven to eleven years. They concluded that those who had undergone surgery for weight loss and lost weight had a 30 percent to 40 percent reduced risk of dying over the next seven to eleven years compared with those without the surgery. Dr. George Bray of the Pennington Biomedical Research Center in Baton Rouge, Louisiana, commented in the same journal, "The question as to whether intentional weight loss improves life span has been answered. The answer appears to be a resounding yes!"

The Genes behind Calorie Restriction

Despite the dramatic study results by McCay in the 1930s, just how calorie restriction worked to increase longevity was still unknown. Over the next five decades, many theories evolved. Dr. Denham Harman, a professor at the University of Nebraska, speculated that dietary restriction reduced energy production in the cells and therefore led to less toxicity from free radicals. That made intuitive sense. Theoretically, fewer free radicals should result in less cellular damage and a longer life. However, antioxidants alone have not been shown to prolong longevity.

Other studies performed on a wide variety of animals showed that calorie restriction enhances the immune response in older animals, thus reducing the onset of fatal age-related diseases. Paradoxically, it seems to impair this system in young animals, and this may be why calorie restriction in children is so dangerous, as in cases of anorexia or in famine-stricken areas of the world. Calorie-restricted monkeys also have decreased triglyceride levels and increased levels of HDL, the good cholesterol, thereby reducing the risk of dying from cardiovascular disease. Calorie restriction also increases insulin sensitivity, allowing the hormone to more effectively control blood sugar and delay adult-onset diabetes, which frequently causes premature death.

But the main action of calorie restriction was to prolong the healthy, disease-free period of life and postpone the period of rapid decline near the end of life. As an added bonus, these studies confirmed that calorie restriction positively affected health even if not started until middle age. It's never too late to start!

Chapter 5

Beginning to Understand Longevity Genes

We and other researchers have found that a family of genes involved in an organism's ability to withstand a stressful environment—such as excessive heat or scarcity of food or water—have the power to keep its natural defense and repair activities going strong, regardless of age.

—DAVID SINCLAIR AND LEONARD GAURENTE, 2007

In the early 1960s, a South African biologist named Sydney Brenner was curious about how genes direct the production of specific proteins. In 1964 he chose the lowly worm *C. elegans* as an experimental model and spent years mapping out just how the 959 cells that make up the worm (compared with our trillions of cells) are generated from the single cell of a worm's egg. As it turned out, the genetic code, even in this very simple organism, was very complex. The code called for numerous enzymes to modify the necessary proteins, as well as for RNA to produce additional molecules essential to the worm's survival. Any alterations in the code or significant changes in environmental conditions would alter the formation of these cells and often lead to the death of the worm. For this work, Sydney Brenner received a Nobel Prize in 2002.

While working on these genetic codes, one of Brenner's students, Cynthia Kenyon, startled the scientific world when she doubled the life span of Brenner's worms by modifying a single gene called daf-2. As Dr. Kenyon put it, before this discovery, "everyone thought aging just happened; to control aging, you had to fix everything, so it was impossible." Her research not only offered a possible explanation for how calorie restriction might work but also suggested an alternative approach to longevity: to control the rate of aging by gaining access to the genetic network that directs cellular activity. Her work amplified the observations of molecular biologists D. B. Friedman and Tom Johnson at the University of California, Irvine, who demonstrated that a single gene mutation was responsible for the enhanced longevity of a strain of worms created in the 1980s by biologist Michael Klass at the University of Houston. This mutation, termed age-1, inspired a raft of research, including Kenyon's work.

From Yeast to Man

What other genetic codes exist that could control aging? And is there a mechanism for aging that works like calorie restriction? Enter Leonard Guarente. In 1981 this brilliant molecular biologist launched his career as an assistant professor at MIT by studying a single basic problem in biology: the regulation of genes and how they get "turned on and off" in cells. After ten years of work, he decided that the new technological tools of the molecular geneticist just might have the power to pinpoint the gene that would turn out to be the holy grail of aging. Intoxicated by this possibility, he made the life-changing decision to study the lowly yeast—the same life-form used to make bread, beer, wine, and various other spirits for thousands of years.

Early on, Guarente and graduate students Brian Kennedy and Nick Austriaco made a seminal observation. After creating a stressful environment for their yeast colonies by reducing the amount of glucose the yeast fed on, the researchers discovered that stressed yeast lived as much as 50 percent longer than yeast given normal quantities of nutrients. Another unusual—and related—observation was that the yeast became sterile under such stress, which mimicked similar reproductive changes that had been seen in Clive McCay's calorie-restricted animals in the 1930s.

The next problem to be solved was whether or not the longevity and sterility were caused by the same genetic mechanism. It turned out that in yeast cells, the SIR4 gene encoded a protein (known as SIR4) that regulated an enzyme called SIR2, which is now famous for its ability to control the life span. SIR2 turns off, or silences, genes in its vicinity, and this fact became a critical element in the antiaging story.

Following the international acclaim generated by his work in age prevention, Dr. Guarente was invited to give seminars all around the world on the genetic aspects of aging. While lecturing at the University of Melbourne in Australia, he decided to visit a friend, Ian Dawes, then chairman of molecular biology at the University of New South Wales in Sydney. Fortuitously, this would lead to the recruitment of a young doctoral student in Dawes's laboratory, David Sinclair. Eventually, through work performed in Guarente's lab, Sinclair would become a star longevity researcher and founder of the Paul F. Glenn Laboratories for the Biological Mechanisms of Aging at Harvard Medical School.

In 1997, two years after arriving at MIT, Sinclair published the first of many papers in the international journal *Cell,* in which he and his mentor, Lenny Guarente, described the cause of aging in yeast. Aging in yeast is measured by counting how many times "mother" cells divide to produce "daughters" before dying. Twenty divisions is a typical yeast cell life span. Investigating why this happens, they discovered that as the mother cells age, a surprising kind of instability occurs in the DNA. After several divisions, a region in the DNA occasionally spins off an extra ring-shaped bit of genetic material before dividing. In subsequent divisions, these rings, like the rest of the genome, are copied, but unlike the rest of the genome, both copies stay in the mother cell. These circular rings continue to accumulate in the mother cell's nucleus and eventually spell her doom (see figure 9).

Next, Sinclair and Guarente discovered that when extra copies of the SIR2 gene were added to the yeast cells, the formation of these abnormal DNA circles slowed down, and the yeast life span was extended

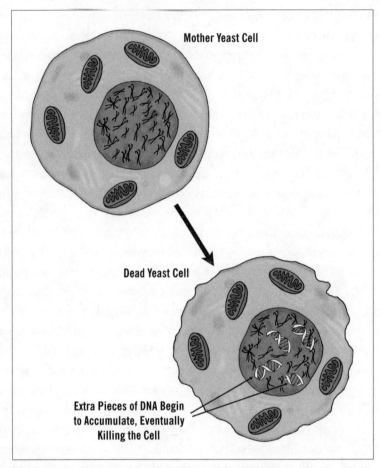

Mother Yeast Cell

Dead Yeast Cell

**Extra Pieces of DNA Begin
to Accumulate, Eventually
Killing the Cell**

FIGURE 9 Excessive residual DNA after approximately 20 cellular
divisions leads to the death of a mother yeast cell.

by 30 percent. They also discovered that the process of forming these
damaging DNA circles could be repressed by reducing the amount of
glucose or amino acids, the building blocks of protein, in the yeast's
nutrients—a treatment akin to calorie restriction in higher organisms.
By doing so, they connected calorie restriction, SIR2 gene activation,
and increased longevity in yeast.

When they began their work, Sinclair and Guarente clearly under-
stood that the very idea that studying the life span of yeast would con-

tribute anything to the knowledge of human aging was considered pre-posterous by many. Yet in these simple experiments, they showed, for the first time, how calorie restriction—and increased longevity—in yeast was related to the function of the SIR2 gene.

These observations had huge implications. They suggested that aging, at least in this model, was not due to "wear and tear," or to the buildup of free radicals due to insufficient antioxidants, or to mutations. Rather, it appeared to be a highly regulated mechanism, which was genetically controlled: SIR2 genes and their enzymes acted in some way to stabilize and ensure proper genetic transfer from one cell to another. Later, when the SIR2 gene was removed from inbred mice, the rodents had significantly shorter lives. Rachel Esposito, a molecular biologist at the University of Chicago, confirmed Sinclair and Guarente's findings. She demonstrated that the SIR2 enzyme enhances the stability of the DNA and suppresses the formation of abnormal DNA.

But how relevant could findings on yeast be to human beings? As the research community pursued the exciting findings of the SIR2 gene in yeast and its mammalian counterpart, *SIRT1*, it became apparent that all living organisms, from bacteria to humans, possess genes for the production of SIR2-like enzymes (dubbed *sirtuins*). By implication, then, this gene complex must play a vital role in all living organisms.

The stage was now set for the next ascent to the Himalayas of longevity: identifying the molecular regulators of sirtuins—and therefore of aging. What was it that turned on the sirtuin genes to do their DNA-stabilizing work? After many elegant experiments, Guarente and his cadre of PhDs investigated two molecules that played key roles in converting glucose and oxygen into the energy necessary for all cellular activity: NAD and NADH. NAD and NADH, molecules present in all living cells, play a critical role in generating energy, as well as many other metabolic processes. Without these substances, cell activity would cease. Guarente postulated that the SIR2 gene could somehow sense when cells became low on energy (or calories), and he connected this information to gene activation. He and his colleagues made the seminal observation that sirtuins require *one* of these molecules, NAD, in order to work, but not the other. They also discovered that during calorie restriction, cellular metabolism shifts to produce more of the sirtuin-friendly molecules, increasing the sirtuins' activity. This, in turn, stabilizes the DNA and slows the formation of the abnormal DNA circles that cause aging—thus slowing the yeast's subsequent death.

A critical connection had been made in the quest to solve the mysteries of aging. To summarize: (1) calorie restriction stresses the organism, directly affecting energy production; (2) an organism under stress has mechanisms within the cell to promote survival until times get better; (3) when cells sense lower levels of energy production, SIR2 enzyme levels rise, creating an environment in the cells that promotes longevity.

Guarente's team published this work in February 2000, setting the stage for the next question about aging: What might be done to activate these specialized longevity genes *without* restricting calories? Was there another way to activate these newly discovered longevity genes directly?

In May 2003 David Sinclair and his lab colleagues Rozalyn Anderson, Kevin Bitterman, Jason Wood, and Oliver Medvedik added another piece to the puzzle with their publication in *Nature*. Just as Guarente and his colleagues had discovered a molecular connection to sirtuin enzymes, Sinclair's team discovered another longevity gene, *PNC1*, which was also activated by restricting calories. This gene, when activated, makes a protein that metabolizes and removes a vitamin B–like compound that normally suppresses, or turns off, SIR2 in yeast cells. If SIR2 is not suppressed, less of it is produced. There are two mechanisms, therefore, through which calorie restriction increases longevity in yeast: increasing the availability of Guarente's molecule, NAD, and activating Sinclair's PNC1 molecule. Both increase SIR2. Both are triggered by calorie restriction, and both increase the SIR2 enzyme's ability to stabilize DNA and extend the yeast life span.

While deciphering how PNC1 governed the life span, Sinclair collaborated with Konrad Howitz, director of molecular biology at Biomol International, a company in Plymouth Meeting, Pennsylvania. They posed another research question: given the evolutionary biology of humans and plants, might there be natural substances or compounds found in our diet that could activate the sirtuin enzymes comparably to activation by caloric restriction or other environmental stressors? This led to other questions: What natural substances would be chosen to test? How could enough SIR2 enzyme be obtained for a test? If done manually, the search for gene activation could take months or longer. What equipment was available for that task?

Fortunately, Howitz had developed several laboratory techniques to evaluate compounds that might activate the SIR2 enzyme or its counterpart in mammals, SIRT1. To their delight, the experiments identified nineteen compounds that stimulated SIRT1 activity, all of which were found in red wine grapes or other plant sources. They referred to these collectively as *sirtuin activating compounds*, or *STACs*. All but two of these STACs were polyphenols, which already were known for their heart and brain protection and cancer-suppression benefits.

What Are Polyphenols?

Polyphenols are the most abundant antioxidants in our diet, and they promote health through a variety of gene activating mechanisms. Polyphenols give the red to red wine, the dark brown to chocolate, and the green to green tea. Grapes, apples, onions, soy, peanuts, berries, and many other fruits and vegetables are loaded with polyphenols.

Phenol, the parent structure of polyphenols, has been used in surgery since the mid-1800s, when Sir Joseph Lister, considered the father of modern surgery, introduced carbolic acid (phenol) to disinfect skin, hands, and surgical instruments to prevent infections. Chemically, the phenol structure is a hexagon of mostly carbon atoms with hydrogen and oxygen attached to one or several of the hexagon's six points. More complex phenols are called "poly" (meaning "many") phenols, because they have several of these hexagons linked together in different configurations.

The essential point is that these small-molecule polyphenolic substances are found naturally in plants and are extremely effective at protecting plants and animals against common health problems and the effects of aging. Plants stressed by drought, infection, ultraviolet radiation from sunlight, and other factors produce even more of these protective polyphenols. Resveratrol, a highly active polyphenol found in high concentrations in the skin of stressed red grapes, is now playing a major role in the antiaging revolution.

Sinclair and Howitz found that resveratrol did indeed increase the life span of yeast by directly stimulating SIR2 activity. For the first time, these investigators found a way to duplicate the benefits of restricted calories with a group of compounds found in red wine and vegetables. In fact, resveratrol extended the yeast life span by up to 60 percent! Even more exciting, the molecules were also active in human cells cultured in the lab. Commenting on the increased life span, Howitz observed, "The sirtuin stimulation provided by certain polyphenols may be a far more important biological effect than their antioxidant action." The brilliant discovery of Howitz and Sinclair demonstrated that by ingesting molecules from stressed plants, animals activate their own "scarcity genes" or "longevity factors," including sirtuins—without needing to suffer caloric restriction.

Sinclair noted: "It can be imagined that throughout evolution, such stress markers found in the xenohormetic molecules [xeno factors] in the surrounding vegetation would have served as strong predictors of a coming drought, famine, or direct stress to the animal. Reacting to these molecules would allow the xenohormetic [stress] response to begin ahead of this severe environmental event to protect against catastrophic damage or energy depletion." Thus plants acted as an early warning system to allow the animal's cellular function to change ahead of an impending stress and promote survival until the stress subsided.

Sinclair stated that several predictions follow from this hypothesis. First, we should find a bounty of medicinal molecules in stressed plants. Second, molecules from stressed plants should be relatively nontoxic, since we evolved along with them. Third, these molecules should interact with the various enzymes and genes involved in regulating longevity.

Following their landmark paper in September 2003 on STACs in yeast, Sinclair and Howitz conducted a study on both worms and flies. The researchers confirmed their prior hypothesis, but with a twist. Unlike sirtuin activation by calorie restriction, which also reduces reproductive capability in animals, the xeno factors found in stressed plants did not reduce reproductive ability in animals. Not only was this a dramatic confirmation of this hypothesis, but it also confirmed that calorie restriction, or starvation, is the crucial indicator as to when an animal species should not reproduce. This makes perfect sense. In times of famine or other harsh conditions, the best strategy would be to focus all available resources on individual survival, deferring reproduction for another time. This strategy presents a clear advantage over competing with offspring for insufficient resources.

How and Why Plants Talk to People

By 2003 scientific answers to the question posed by Clive McCay seventy years earlier—"Why does calorie restriction increase longevity?"—were finally forthcoming from studies on the biologically ancient yeast and worms. The discovery of longevity genes, how they are activated, and the biochemical mechanisms they rely on to increase longevity and enhance health was a scientific coup. The further discovery that specific plant molecules found in our food supply can activate longevity genes without calorie restriction has become the domain of a whole new scientific area of investigation called nutrigenomics. This science studies the mechanisms by which specific foods activate our genes: for instance, how trans fats in French fries turn on genes that raise our "bad" cholesterol, and how resveratrol, tea, soy, and thousands of other polyphenols protect our health.

The concept of food as fuel only no longer holds. Even the simplest foods contain hundreds of specialized molecules. Some are nutritive (providing energy), but others are bioactive, capable of effecting changes in hormone levels and in fat, carbohydrate, and protein metabolism. This plant-to-animal interaction is as ancient as humankind itself. Twenty-five percent of our prescription drugs and nearly all of our recreational chemical substances are plant derived. This figure includes the caffeine in coffee, the nicotine in tobacco, the theophylline in tea, and the theobromine in chocolate, not to mention the addictive drugs marijuana, cocaine, and more. All are part of this ancient plant-animal interaction. Howitz and Sinclair beautifully summarized this in their May 2008 article in *Cell,* "Xenohormesis: Sensing the Chemical Cues of Other Species."

The concept of xenohormesis asserts that certain molecules in our food can have significant health- and longevity-enhancing effects that may turn out to surpass anything current medications can achieve. This would not have come as news to Hippocrates, the father of Western medicine, who said, "Let food be your medicine and medicine be your food."

Chapter 6

The French Paradox and the Holy Grail of Aging

No matter what field you are in, if you are working outside the box, perseverance, tenacity, stubbornness, and curiosity is what is required to overcome certain failure.

—GEORGE LUCAS, AMERICAN FILM DIRECTOR,
PRODUCER, AND SCREENWRITER, 2007

In moderate amount, wine is the best medicine for soul and body.

—VOLTAIRE, FRENCH PHILOSOPHER, 1694–1778

On November 17, 1991, the CBS TV program *60 Minutes* broadcast a story suggesting that French people's consumption of red wine was the reason for the lower rate of heart disease in France. The report noted that the French ate almost 40 percent more grams of fat from animal sources per day than Americans, as well as four times as much butter, 60 percent more cheese, and nearly three times more pork. Yet in France the death rate from heart attacks was half what it was in the United States.

The broadcast suggested that France's high red wine consumption was responsible for this counterintuitive notion, which was called the "French paradox." During the four weeks following the broadcast, U.S. supermarkets and liquor stores recorded a 44 percent increase in the sale of red wine.

Fast-forward twelve years. By 2003, sirtuin genes were emerging as key mediators of the effects of caloric restriction, which improves the metabolism of carbohydrates and fat—both excessive in the French diet. Was it therefore possible that sirtuin genes might play a role in the French paradox? But the French *weren't* starving. How did resveratrol and the other polyphenols in red wine lower cardiovascular risk in the French? Was it the antioxidant effects of these polyphenols?

It is now generally agreed that red wines contain the polyphenols known as *resveratrol, quercetin, catechins,* and others, all of which have powerful beneficial biological activities, including prevention of heart attacks, cancer, and strokes. The 2003 paper by Howitz and Sinclair confirmed that resveratrol and other xeno factors activated the SIRT1 gene, so the French paradox appeared to have been solved. According to this xenohormesis hypothesis, these small molecules found in red wine can activate the sirtuin gene—in the absence of calorie restriction—to provide the same cardio-protective benefits as wine, without the alcohol. Thanks to the science of ethnobotany, which studies how and why different cultures use plants, and nutrigenomics, we now had the best explanation for the French paradox.

Xeno factors like resveratrol, the most potent polyphenol SIRT1 activator, are found in abundance not only in red grape skins and concentrated red wine and grape juice, but also in the root of a very interesting plant called giant knotweed, or *hu zhang,* used for centuries by the Chinese and Japanese for its health benefits. Smaller concentrations are found in peanuts, dark chocolate, and various berries (see table 2). Resveratrol is in the subgroup of polyphenols known as *stilbenes* and is also classified as a *phytoalexin,* meaning a stress-induced molecule in plants with antifungal activity and other defensive properties. This is consistent with the fact that grapes with the highest resveratrol content are found in humid, cool locations where fungus is most common. Winegrowers know this and strategically place vineyards all over the world in these locations.

Another paradox is that resveratrol is found in relatively low concentration in red wine—approximately 1 milligram (mg) to 5 milligrams per liter, although there is considerable variation depending

TABLE 2 Dietary Sources of Resveratrol

Red wine	Peanuts
White wine	Roasted peanuts
Port and sherry	Boiled peanuts
Grapes	Peanut butter
Dry grape skins	100 percent natural peanut butter
Red grape juice	Pistachios
White grape juice	Hops
Raw cranberry juice	Giant knotweed (*Polygonum cuspidatum*)
Blueberries	Dry rhubarb root
Billberries	Pomegranate juice
Lingonberries	Dark chocolate

on the type of grape and how and where it is grown. Part of the health benefit, therefore, may be the additive or even synergistic effects between resveratrol and other wine polyphenols, including those that provide the color pigment of grapes. Resveratrol itself is colorless, and also is present in white grape skins, but not in high concentration, because white grape skins are generally not soaked with wine juice for the same duration as the skins used in making red wines. As a group, the polyphenols found in the skin of red wine grapes are the most abundant polyphenols in red wine—up to 1 gram per liter in some organically grown red wines. Research on this polyphenol has also revealed protection in major blood vessels from plaque formation, or hardening of the arteries.

Recent studies reviewing the concentrations of resveratrol in red wines demonstrate that the amount seems to be too low to completely explain the French paradox. One reason may be the widespread use of herbicides and pesticides on grapes to increase yields.

These unstressed grape skins produce low amounts of the defensive phytoalexins, reducing their concentration in the wine. Organically grown wine and vintage bottles forty or fifty years old may have two to five times more xeno factors in them, because no pesticides or chemicals are used on them during their growth. Professor Roger Corder at the William Harvey Research Institute in London has identified another group of polyphenols, *oligomeric procyanidins*, which are also found in high levels in red grape skins. He reports that in addition to protecting human blood vessels, these compounds may play a role in lowering blood pressure.

What's a Fish Got to Do with It?

Howitz and Sinclair's publication in *Nature* solidified the new paradigm in aging research developing since the early 1990s. Now it was possible to directly affect the regulators of aging with natural food-based substances. The scientific world would confirm these findings, and soon Sinclair and his associates were looking up the evolutionary biological ladder to the vertebrates. Could scientific observations in lower organisms (namely yeast, roundworms, and fruit flies) be confirmed in animals with backbones, such as fish, amphibians, reptiles, birds, and mammals? The answer was yes, but this story of discovery takes many turns, and we must first learn more about how special creatures such as the African turquoise killifish, with its maximum life span of only twelve weeks, contributed to understanding the French paradox and longevity.

Scientists who study longevity are constantly on the lookout for creatures with a very short natural life span, or "shortevity." This allows researchers to manipulate the cycle of life and death in a cost-effective manner, and it is why Lenny Guarente and his MIT graduate students zeroed in on the lowly yeast. They subsequently moved up to the roundworm, which diverged from the yeast several hundred million years ago. When they found the same gene in both organisms, they speculated that it might be shared with other animals, including humans. Then came the work out of Guarente's lab, and later at Sinclair's lab, showing that the activation of sirtuin enzymes required the presence of another molecule involved in numerous metabolic reactions—

energy production in particular. "This finding meant to us that sirtuins could connect aging to metabolism [not just to DNA] and therefore to diet, since food provides our energy fuel," said Guarente. "Once you see this activity, a child could point out that maybe this would connect to calorie restriction."

The identification of xeno factors that could actually activate the sirtuins astounded longevity scientists, and opened up the possibility of developing drugs that could interact with sirtuins and turn on their beneficial effects. But could the plant-based polyphenols discovered by Sinclair be used to accomplish the same end? With the foundation established first in yeast and flatworms, it was time for Italian researchers to make a major contribution to the puzzle of life and longevity, using the two-inch-long turquoise killifish found in tsetse fly–infested seasonal pools in Zimbabwe and Mozambique. In 2005 Dr. Dario Valenzano and his colleagues in Pisa conceived an experiment to determine if resveratrol could slow the onset of aging in this vertebrate.

Dr. Valenzano took 157 turquoise killifish—which age approximately five hundred times faster than we do—and added resveratrol to their diet in three different concentrations: 24 micrograms (mcg), 120 micrograms, and 600 micrograms of resveratrol per gram of food. A fourth group was used as a control and received no resveratrol.

The results of this study, published in November 2006 in the journal *Current Biology,* astonished the scientific community: all of the control fish died by the expected twelve weeks of age, as did the fish receiving the lowest dose of resveratrol. The fish receiving the two higher doses not only lived much longer, but did so in a dose-dependent fashion: the group given 120 micrograms lived 27 percent longer, and the highest dose increased longevity by an astounding 59 percent. Another major observation was no loss of fertility, as occurs with caloric restriction in mammals; on the contrary, the resveratrol-fed females continued to lay eggs that were fertilized by the resveratrol-fed males beyond the twelve weeks that were the expected age of death. In addition, the eggs hatched normally, and the offspring developed into normal adults.

Prompted by observations from Guarente's and Sinclair's labs, the

Italian scientists also measured the fishes' swimming activity, using an automated video tracking system that constantly monitored the location of each fish in the tank. They analyzed average swimming speed and time spent moving. By nine weeks, the control fish were slower in all major categories. In contrast, resveratrol-fed fish increased their swimming activity by up to one-third.

Next the Italian researchers wanted to see if the longer-lived fish lost brain capabilities as they aged. How do you measure brain function in a fish? Valenzano and his colleagues trained fish to avoid a certain stimulus: a red light in the tank. They were able to demonstrate that resveratrol-supplemented fish avoided the information-processing decline seen in control fish as they aged. When they examined brain cells of the control fish and those of resveratrol-treated fish, they found in the older control group degeneration comparable to human Alzheimer's. The cells of the older treated fish showed no evidence of this.

The experiment was an unequivocal demonstration of increased longevity, as well as major protection of muscle and brain functions. The implications represented another giant step up the evolutionary tree and set the stage for the next blockbuster discovery.

The Paradox of a High-Fat, High-Calorie Diet and Normal Weight

While the Italian investigators were studying their vertebrate fish, David Sinclair had already begun conducting experiments for the next major breakthrough in aging—in mammals this time. By now he was well known as one of the major players in this emerging field of longevity and genes. As Sinclair's recognition grew, so did the number of postdoctoral applicants wanting to join his lab at Harvard. In 2003 Joseph Baur had just completed his PhD in integrative biology, having already been an author and coauthor of several articles on life extension. After a short interview, Sinclair hired Baur to lead the mammal research project.

Building upon the brilliant scientific discoveries of Mendel, Darwin, Watson and Crick, Kenyon, Guarente, and Sinclair himself, Sinclair and Baur methodically studied, planned, and then executed the next coup in longevity research.

They knew that reducing calorie intake by approximately 40 percent was the most reproducible and effective way to delay age-related diseases and extend the life span in mammals. They also knew that the sirtuin genes and the enzymes they produce in mammals regulated such processes as glucose and insulin production, fat metabolism, and cell survival, and that these actions might be responsible for the benefits of caloric restriction. The next step would be to try to mimic those benefits using an outside stimulus. After screening more than twenty thousand molecules and identifying the major natural xeno factor compounds (produced in abundance in a relatively small number of stressed plants), they were ready.

To carry out their study, Sinclair and Baur enlisted the help of Rafael de Cabo, an investigator at the National Institute on Aging's scientific laboratories in Bethesda, Maryland, and expert on calorie restriction in rodents. Although de Cabo was initially dubious in the face of their excitement, a sample of resveratrol quickly changed his mind. After seeing tumors in some of his mice reduced tenfold, de Cabo called back and demanded, "What is this stuff?" The addition of Kevin Pearson, an energetic young scientist who had just completed his PhD at the University of Cincinnati, rounded out the core group.

The Harvard experiment was simple and elegant. It involved three groups of middle-aged (one-year-old) male mice. One group was given a standard diet; the second group was given an otherwise equivalent but high-calorie, high-fat diet; and the third group was fed the same high-calorie, high-fat diet as the second group, but this time with resveratrol, at two different concentrations.

The study, published on November 1, 2006, in the journal *Nature,* resonated around the world. Dr. Sinclair's findings made the front page of the *Wall Street Journal*, the *New York Times*, the *Washington Post,* and *Newsweek*—even Russia's *Pravda*—and appeared on most television stations around the world. In answer to "Can you have your cake and eat it too?" the answer seemed to be a resounding yes; for the first time, a xeno factor, resveratrol, was found to offset the bad health effects of a high-calorie diet and to significantly extend the life span.

Obesity is now a worldwide epidemic. In obese or overweight people, the major complication of high-calorie, high-fat diets is an increase in glucose and insulin levels that often leads to diabetes, cardiovascular disease, and fatty deposits in the liver. These same effects were observed in the mice fed a high-calorie diet. Conversely, however, the high-calorie resveratrol group had significantly lower levels of glucose, insulin, and other markers of diabetes. Although the mice still gained weight, their tendency toward diabetes and other age-related diseases was reduced. The lower insulin levels also predicted increased life span. Moreover, the resveratrol-treated mice showed improved balance and motor coordination, reminiscent of the positive swimming results in the killifish experiment.

The researchers took the study one step further and examined microscopically the tested animals' hearts, livers, and various other tissues. Whereas the liver and heart in the high-calorie-fed animals exhibited a loss of cellular integrity and a buildup of fat, the high-calorie-plus-resveratrol group appeared normal and healthy. In addition, the liver cells showed increased numbers of mitochondria, indicating an enhanced ability to metabolize glucose and fat.

In a similar study in the lab of Johan Auwerx at the Institute of Genetics and Molecular and Cellular Biology in France, resveratrol again improved insulin sensitivity and motor coordination in mice. These researchers, however, focused primarily on muscle tissue and were able to show a dramatic increase in aerobic capacity and endurance in the treated mice. These impressive results appear to be attributable to an increase in the number of mitochondria in muscle tissue. Additionally, with the higher doses employed by Auwerx's group, the mice did not gain weight despite a high-calorie diet. Baur summarized these results by stating, "This work demonstrates that there may be tremendous medical benefits to unlocking the secrets behind the genes that control our longevity. No doubt many more remain to be discovered in the coming years."

Indeed, following their landmark 2006 report showing that resveratrol improves health and longevity in overweight aged mice, Rafael de Cabo and David Sinclair began planning their next research coup. For this they enlisted the help of an international group of researchers and obtained funding from the National Institute on Aging. They fed mice a standard diet, a high-calorie diet, or an every-other-day feeding regimen, each one with and without resveratrol. In the resveratrol-treated group, they found a dramatic decrease in heart and blood vessel disease, a decrease in cholesterol levels, stronger and thicker bones, and an increased life span in those mice fed a high-calorie diet. They reported these dramatic findings in July 2008 in the journal *Cell Metabolism*. The director of the National Institutes of Health, Richard Hodes, MD, commented, "Resveratrol has produced significant effects in animal models, now including mice, where it mimics some, but not all, consequences of caloric restriction."

In summary, resveratrol demonstrated the following benefits in animal studies:

- Despite a high-fat diet, the treated mice *did not gain weight* and had smaller fat cells.
- It protected the animals from developing a diabetes-like condition.
- It increased the number of energy-producing mitochondria in muscle cells—without additional exercise!
- It boosted the burning of body fat.
- It increased the aerobic capacity (endurance) of the mice when tested on treadmills.
- It maintained their cell sensitivity to insulin, moderating blood sugar levels.
- It transformed muscle fibers into the slow type seen in trained athletes—again, without training.
- It enhanced muscle strength and reduced muscle fatigue.
- It improved the animals' coordination.
- There were no adverse affects on the liver or other organ cells.

This research set off a wave of new studies, many of which have focused on polyphenols' ability to make significant breakthroughs in the treatment of—and prevention of—most of the major diseases that threaten humankind. We will explore this stunning series of developments in the chapters ahead, but first we digress to pursue an exceedingly practical question: can these miracle polyphenols be packaged and produced commercially so they can be available for all of us?

Part II

The Australian Extract

Chapter 7

Serendipity and the Australian Connection

I once read a silly fairy tale called "The Three Princes of Serendip." As their highnesses traveled, they were always making discoveries, by accident and sagacity, of things which they were not in quest of.

—HORACE WALPOLE

Serendipity—accidentally discovering something fortunate, especially while looking for something else entirely—is a major component of scientific discovery and invention. Scottish biologist Alexander Fleming failed to disinfect cultures of bacteria when leaving for his vacation; on his return, he found them contaminated with penicillium mold, which killed the bacteria. A Peruvian Indian discovered quinine during a malarial attack by drinking water in a pool under a cinchona tree; the fever abated, and a Jesuit priest who heard the story popularized cinchona bark by sharing it with infected clerics in Rome. The final link in the discovery of DNA occurred when Francis Crick serendipitously glanced at Rosalind Franklin's careful X-ray measurements in a report he was not supposed to see and, in a flash of insight, saw the double-coiled helix in his mind.

The British politician and writer Horace Walpole coined the word *serendipity* in a letter dated January 28, 1754, to describe the accidental and unexpected discovery of something of a positive nature. Walpole derived the word from a fairy tale, "The Three Princes of Serendip," in which three traveling princes stumbled across wonderful things entirely by chance. Serendip, later called Ceylon and now known as Sri Lanka, is the lushly overgrown island that is described as hanging like a pearl from India's southern tip.

We've seen serendipity at work in our story of yeast, worms, and mice in the laboratories of David Sinclair and Lenny Guarente. But equally serendipitous was a discovery that took place far from any clinical setting: in a vineyard in the fertile hills of Australia's Mornington Peninsula. "The Peninsula," as it is known, is an uncharacteristically green corner of an arid continent. Its beaches are playgrounds for well-to-do families from nearby Melbourne, and its temperate hinterland is home to dozens of vineyards that produce some of Australia's finest wine grapes. It is a cool, moist region renowned for its long, slow ripening periods. The grape harvest often takes place as late as April, well into the Southern Hemisphere's autumn.

On an April Sunday in 2004, Peter Voigt and his wife, Lynda Field, called on a small army of friends to help pick wine grapes from their diminutive estate in the Peninsula hills. The weather was far from idyllic, but there was much camaraderie among the warmly clad pickers as they trudged through mist and drizzle. The Voigts were certainly not complaining. More than anything, they felt relieved to have a grape crop to harvest at all that year.

Neither was a professional winemaker. Peter was a biochemist turned businessman, the energetic CEO of a successful and innovative company that specialized in sustainable solutions to engineering challenges. He'd met American-born Lynda while on business in the United States, and they shared, among many things, a love of fine wine. In 2002 they bought one of the Mornington Peninsula's most beautiful and best-regarded vineyards, high on a hill near a dramatic coastal escarpment.

In theory it made perfect sense: The lush setting, only an hour's drive from their company headquarters, was stunning. Wine from the vineyard's grapes had won international prizes. Cash flow seemed guaranteed, since one of the region's best wineries had contracted to buy the estate's grapes. But within weeks of moving in, the Voigts came to the unhappy realization that owning a vineyard involved more business than pleasure, and that their vineyard demanded more work than most. One factor was the weather. The Peninsula's maritime climate is known for its humidity, and the Voigt vineyard was a haven for fungal infections. Plus, the vineyard was planted for Pinot Noir, a thin-skinned red grape variety that grows in tightly clustered bunches. Known in the wine industry as "the heartbreak grape" for its charm, fickle temperament, and low yields, Pinot Noir is a perfect habitat for fungal growth. Making prizewinning wines from this vineyard, the Voigts were told, depended on regular prophylactic spraying with antifungal agents and pesticides.

Peter found himself spending his days at the office—where he developed environmentally friendly technologies for controlling air pollution and water treatment—and then, at night, spending hours on his aging tractor, spraying the vineyard with toxic chemicals. The irony was not lost on him, and the tedious hours at the wheel gave him plenty of time to think. Increasingly, he was thinking that conventional winegrowing practice was wrong. Chemical warfare, he thought, not only was ruinously expensive and labor intensive but seemed at odds with making a beverage that was supposed to be a reflection of its environment.

Peter's research led him to understand that his red grapes had their own defensive response to threats such as stress, UV light, and fungal diseases. When under attack, he learned, the red grape produces antifungal compounds known as phytoalexins. The grape concentrates these compounds in its skin, the front line of defense. These polyphenol phytoalexins, as discussed earlier, have been implicated in the French paradox as protectors of the heart and blood vessels.

Peter Voigt reasoned that if he minimized antifungal spraying and stressed his vines by not pruning and by allowing all the grape bunches to ripen, the grapes would produce their own defenses. Not only would this save him time and money, but encouraging the development of these defensive compounds might result in especially polyphenol-rich wine.

Unbeknownst to Voigt this process had been previously demonstrated by Langcake and Pryce in 1976. They had also concluded that with highly infected fruit there would be higher resveratrol levels in the wine. But they also showed that resveratrol levels decrease with very high levels of fungus infection. The authors believed that a fungal enzyme, if present in too large of an amount in the wine juice, may actually degrade resveratrol in the final wine product. Although resveratrol levels were found in wine with no infection, the highest levels of resveratrol were in wines made with grapes with approximately 10 percent infection.

Peter began to roll out his plan in the spring of 2003 by spraying against fungus only when infection occurred. Experienced winegrowers shook their heads and told him this could cost him his entire crop if infection took hold. Eyebrows were raised a few months later when Peter declined to "thin" the fruit on his vines—a preharvest practice of snipping off a percentage of grape bunches to aid the quality of those that remain. Peter wanted the vines to carry as much fruit as possible in hopes of triggering a stress response would protect his grapes naturally.

It was an unconventional, high-risk approach to growing this most temperamental of grape varieties, and the winemaker to whom the Voigts had agreed to sell their crop was not happy. He warned that even if the grapes survived the growing season without succumbing to disease, there was a chance that the vines would be too burdened with fruit for the grapes to develop the proper flavor.

By harvesttime in 2004, Peter had nearly lost his crop to infection more than once, and his maverick ways had almost cost him his grape buyer. As it was, the buyer was prepared to take only some of the grapes the Voigts had grown. Those grapes were excellent and became an acclaimed Pinot Noir, but at the time, a worldwide wine glut was under way. Buyers no longer clamored for premium, hand-reared Pinot Noir and Chardonnay. As a result, sensible growers with excess grapes let them rot on the vine. But Peter had not come this far to quit. His vineyard experiment had worked: the grapes were in good condition, and there were plenty of them. He decided to make the wine himself.

Within days of the harvest, the Pinot Noir juice was sitting in tanks in the tractor shed, fermenting on its skins. Later that year, the Voigts pressed out their Pinot before moving it into oak barrels. Peter, the first-time winemaker, was struck by the sheer volume of leftover skins and seeds. So much waste! His past work in food science prompted him to wonder if there was anything of value in this stuff—especially the skins—after all the risks he'd taken to crank up their polyphenol phytoalexin content.

Peter decided to find out. The skins, which had been only lightly pressed, went back into the tank with plenty of juice. He topped the tank with rainwater and installed a pump. For the next four weeks, it ran three times a day, circulating the skins through the liquid, just as it had done for the wine. At the same time, he stepped up his research, this time focusing on how and why chemicals in grape skins were produced.

While Peter's knowledge grew, the brew out in his shed grew darker and more intense. By the end of those four weeks, the liquid was as dark as his Pinot Noir wine had been, supporting Peter's notion that the original Pinot ferment had extracted only half of the skins' contents. He had more than a hunch that this liquid contained something valuable, and, in another instance of serendipity, he just happened to have the means of finding out.

A research team at Peter's company, Clean TeQ, had been reporting exciting results from new separation and purification technologies that could selectively separate out certain chemicals and molecules from a liquid source and concentrate them. Here was an excellent opportunity to get the guys in research and development (R&D) to work on his brew of grape skins, wine, and water. Peter transferred the liquid into containers, loaded them onto the back of a truck, and drove them to his offices in an industrial area of Melbourne, where his researchers assembled their extraction equipment and put it to work on the liquid. They set up a column using beads of an absorbent resin capable of extracting the xeno factors found in red grape skins.

As the liquid was pumped into the column, Peter and the team looked on expectantly. They processed 1,000 liters of the liquid and ended up with ten liters of a thick, dark substance stuck to the beads. It proved to be an intensely purple syrup with a honeylike consistency. This, Peter believed, contained all the polyphenols and phytoalexins— both of which he had read about in David Sinclair's 2003 article in *Nature.*

Peter knew he had something special but was uncertain about his next step. Over the following twelve months, he consumed a teaspoon (5 milliliters) of the extract daily with his breakfast yogurt, hoping that he would suffer no ill effects. He felt fine—better, even—and in every spare moment, he continued to read. One name that emerged again and again was that of Dr. David Sinclair, director of the antiaging laboratory at Harvard Medical School. Feeling a bit tentative, Voigt emailed the renowned researcher, explaining what he had been doing. To his astonishment, he received a reply within the hour: the Harvard professor wanted to know more.

The two men arranged to courier a sample of the extract to Harvard. Lab analysis showed that Voigt's extraction technique had produced an extraordinary concentration of natural polyphenols. This blend would allow for better absorption, reasoned Sinclair, as seen with red wine, yet would contain levels of healthful xeno factors hundreds of times more concentrated than those found in wine. It would be a "superwine," without the alcohol.

The brilliant Harvard professor and the resourceful biochemical engineer met for the first time in November 2005 and found that they were strongly connected. In addition to their Australian upbringing, both men were determined, creative, insightful, and unconventional. Both were amazed to discover that they had each been working to the same end—Sinclair from the theoretical perspective and Voigt from a practical one. With their shared penchant for Australian wine and late-night conversation, they became fast friends.

The two men agreed to work together to determine whether Voigt's Australian extract could activate the SIRT1 survival enzyme. Laboratory analysis revealed that giving the Australian extract to yeast cells resulted in as large an increase in longevity as was seen with resveratrol. And in a second analysis, in which additional pure res-

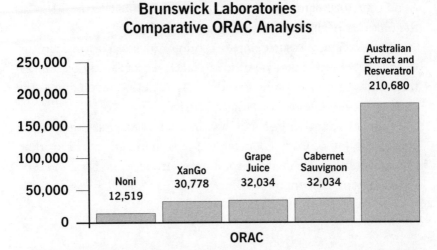

Brunswick Laboratories
Comparative ORAC Analysis

The ORAC (oxygen radical absorbance capacity) analysis provides a measure of the scavenging capacity of antioxidants against the peroxyl rtadical, which is one of the most common reactive oxygen species (ROS) found in the body. ORAC reflects total antioxidant capacity.

The acceptable precision of the ORAC assay is 15 percent relative standard deviation. Testing performed by J. Frietas and J. Theobald, 12/20/2006.

Note: Brunswick Laboratories is used by the USDA for its comparative analyses.

FIGURE 10 Comparison of antioxidant levels of two brand-name mixed fruit juices, grape juice, wine, and a mixture of resveratrol and the Australian extract.

veratrol was added to the extract, no greater longevity was seen. This, they believed, was due to maximal SIR2 enzyme activation by the natural extract, thanks to bioactive polyphenol compounds such as quercetin, fisetin, resveratrol, and others in this brew of concentrated polyphenols working together. Peter Voigt's vineyard travails had led him to serendipitously discover a natural polyphenol cocktail of potent phytoalexins that appeared to work in a lab every bit as well as pharmaceutical-grade resveratrol.

Little did Peter Voigt know at the time that others around the world were also inspired by the research done at Harvard, MIT, and labs in France and that the race was on to develop new natural sources of polyphenols that might be sold to a waiting public anxious to reap the reported health benefits.

The next study was to compare the antioxidant capacity of the Australian extract with that of grape juice and Cabernet Sauvignon. The extract and resveratrol were found to have nearly seven times the antioxidant and free-radical-savaging capacity.

Now the question became: how might this Australian grape skin cocktail or any similarly concentrated polyphenolic mixture work in humans? Might it also increase endurance, strength, memory, and even longevity?

Chapter 8

Leaps of Faith

Every noble work is at first impossible.

—THOMAS CARLYLE

*In all human affairs, there are efforts and there are results,
and the strength of the effort is the measure of the result.*

—JAMES ALLEN

By March 2006 Peter Voigt's wine-making neighbors on Australia's Mornington Peninsula were certain that the man was a few cards short of a full deck. First there had been the peculiar matter of "stressing" his vineyard—deliberately exposing his grapes to disease—and almost losing his crop. Then there was that business of brewing up a vat of red grape skins and water. Surely the man was unhinged. Now, unbelievably, he had turned garbage collector! Most of the district's many wineries paid contractors to remove the huge piles of grape "marc"— the debris of stems and skins—left over after the annual wine crush. But Peter had contacted every winery for miles around and offered to take the waste off their hands for nothing. What on earth, they wondered, did Peter Voigt think he was he doing?

Voigt's late-night discussions with Harvard's Dr. David Sinclair had left him with no doubt that a superconcentrated grape skin Australian extract had the potential to offer extraordinary health benefits. Was it possible, he wondered, to produce the extract in commercial quantities? Using the same process that had worked so well with his first batch, Voigt dramatically scaled up his resin extraction techniques and moved his operations from his vineyard to a local plant designed originally to extract residual red wine juice from already pressed grape skins from the wineries in southern Australia.

It was a turning point. Now Voigt knew with certainty that the project he had begun in his tractor shed back in 2003 had moved beyond being a personal obsession. It had taken on a momentum of its own. He was about to need a lot of money, and soon. He would need to persuade financiers to make a leap of faith, and he would have to find a market, fast.

From Extract to Product

After several conversations with David Sinclair, I became personally convinced of the potential, remarkable health benefits of concentrated polyphenols found in grape skins like the Australian extract and resveratrol. Aware that pharmaceutical companies such as Elixir and Sirtris had been formed to manufacture pharmaceutical-grade resveratrol products, I knew that it would be seven to ten years before these would be available. Furthermore, scientists like Sinclair, and others most involved with the research work, were themselves taking daily doses of purified resveratrol supplements for their health benefits, which seemed to me to be another good sign.

In October 2006, over a glass of red wine, I recounted the story of David Sinclair and Peter Voigt to my good friend David Sculley. Sculley was the president and CEO of the H. J. Heinz Company in Pittsburgh, and now is chairman of the Wedgwood and Royal Doulton companies in the U.K. He immediately called his friend and colleague Bill Watts to tell him of the amazing recent discoveries in the field of longevity and endurance. Watts was the former CEO of General Nutrition Corporation (GNC), the largest supplement company in the United States. These two men both became impressed with the science and also the potential of a marketable product that could be developed from concentrated xeno factors. After further conversations, they formed a company to acquire the patent rights on xenohormetic molecules from Harvard University, procure the plant xeno factors, and make them available to the public. When Harvard University endorsed the venture, Xenomis became the first nutraceutical company to be licensed a Harvard patent. The patent, based on the work of Harvard's David Sinclair, provides Harvard with equity derived from any sales and Xenomis a degree of protection for its products if and when they are developed and marketed.

Because of the potential blockbuster nature of such a product, Xenomis will require a high-volume source of concentrated red grapes to supply the xeno factor products. Several national and international sources, including those produced by Peter Voigt in Australia, may be needed for such a venture.

It had been four years since Peter Voigt had embarked on his crazy plan to subject his vineyard to a high-stress regimen. That had been the first of many leaps of faith on his part, when he had backed his own judgment in spite of the many setbacks and costs. Since that time, a number of other start-up as well as established companies have recognized the tremendous potential to market concentrated xeno factors and have begun producing grape skin concentrates. One of the most significant is a concentrate from the muscadine grape.

Muscadine Grapes

Muscadine grapes (*V. rotundifolia*) are native to North America and may be the only fruit that originated in the United States and nowhere else. They grow almost exclusively in the southeastern United States, primarily in Georgia, South Carolina, Florida, and Alabama. They thrive under adverse conditions perhaps due to their thicker and tougher skin compared to European grapes (*V. vinifera*). Perhaps one reason for these differences in species of grapes, according to geneticists, is that muscadines have an extra chromosome (twenty instead of the nineteen that other grapes have). These additional genes allow muscadine grapes to produce a unique phytochemical, ellagic acid. The ellagic acid polyphenol compounds that are in muscadine grapes are virtually absent in other grapes. Ellagic acid is used by the muscadine grape skin to make tannin called ellagotannins, which is used as an antimicrobial by the plant. Ellagic acid also has powerful antioxidant and anticancer properties. Specifically, studies on cancer cell cultures of the breast, pancreas, esophagus, skin, colon, and prostate demonstrate ellagic acid possesses important anticancer activity. Recently, research in investigating the anticancer effects of muscadine extracts in numerous animal species including man has been initiated.

Additionally, the polyphenols in muscadine grape skins have been shown to have positive effects on heart disease, high cholesterol, diabetes, metabolic syndrome, and other inflammatory conditions. One of the more interesting effects of muscadine products, as well as other grape-derived polyphenol products, appears to be their inhibition of AGE protein formation. As mentioned, these sugar bound proteins can wreak havoc in diabetics and prediabetics and cause complications involving the eye, kidneys, nerves, and blood vessels. Muscadine extracts specifically have been shown to inhibit the release of harmful cytokines, including NF-κB, a master regulator of the inflammatory response.

This species of grape, as shown in some studies, may have a higher resveratrol content than the European grape (*V. vinifera*) that is currently used to make most commercial wines sold around the world. Additional studies indicate muscadines have a higher ORAC value as well. We will provide a table in a later chapter indicating a Xeno score in which we list black grapes, including muscadine grapes, as having a Xeno score of 5—the highest level of resveratrol. There are a number of jams, jellies, and juices made from the muscadine grape that continue to increase in popularity and are specifically marketed as an alcohol-free way to consume natural polyphenol containing products. Muscadine grapes are also made into wines, though they have not become overly popular.

Recently, a large nutrition, direct-selling company, Shaklee Corporation, working with scientists from the University of Georgia, has created a product containing an extract made from muscadine pomace, which is the remaining fruit solids after the water content is extracted.

Specifically they are working with muscadine grape growers in order to secure grapes with large amounts of protective polyphenols including ellagic acid and resveratrol. By selecting local muscadine grapes and by using a whole grape extraction process they have reported that their extract has a significantly higher concentration of healthy polyphenols than found in the skins themselves. A review of their product is found in a later chapter.

Part III

Health Benefits of Xeno Factors

Chapter 9

Live Longer, Improve Memory, Enhance Endurance, and More

In mammals, there is a growing evidence that resveratrol can prevent or delay the onset of cancer, heart disease, ischemic and chemically induced injuries, diabetes, pathological inflammation, and viral infection.

—JOSEPH A. BAUR AND DAVID SINCLAIR,
HARVARD UNIVERSITY, 2006

Since earliest recorded history, humankind has sought to prolong life. According to Greek mythology, Tithonus tricked the gods into granting him immortality. Once they realized their error, the gods withheld eternal youth, and Tithonus was doomed to spend all of eternity getting older and more decrepit. Finally the pathos was too much, even for the notoriously cruel Olympian gods, and they turned him into a grasshopper. Also in Greek mythology, the sibyl of Cumae asked Apollo for immortality but similarly forgot to ask for eternal youth. She grew so old and shrunken that she was put into a jar and eventually became just a voice. From the myths of ancient Greece to Ponce de León's quest for the fountain of youth to the thriving plastic surgery clinics throughout the world today, the search for longevity, vitality, and a youthful appearance goes on.

In the early and middle stages of my medical career, my focus was on acquiring the surgical skills to be able to cure some of the diseases

of aging, such as brain and spinal tumors, and degenerative and ruptured disks in the spine. In cases where surgery couldn't correct the
underlying problem, I would perform various operations intended to
relieve painful symptoms. With time and experience, however, I have
come to realize the importance of preventive medicine. How much
better it would be to prevent disease and improve health in later life
rather than to prolong, at times, misery, and even dying. How much
better it would be to help people stay in relatively good health until
death came. It was Hippocrates, the father of Western medicine, who
summed up this philosophy in his later years by writing, "The first re-
sponsibility of a physician is to prevent disease. If that be impossible,
to cure it. If that too be impossible, then relieve pain."

Dr. Ronald Klatz, cofounder of the American Academy of Anti-
Aging Medicine, which now has more than fifty thousand professional
members, put it another way: "Antiaging or preventive medicine is not
about stretching out the last years of life. It's about stretching out the
middle years of life . . . and actually compressing those last few years of
life so that diseases of aging happen very, very late in the life cycle, just
before death, or don't happen at all."

Lenny Guarente, guru of the science of living longer, said, "The research that I'm involved in is not about extending life after people are
infirm. I don't think of life span as the gold standard. The gold standard is *health* span . . . If you can extend health span, and you also happen to extend life span, so be it." This is the essence of enlightened
preventive medicine and the purpose of this book.

To Live Longer

In the last hundred years, the causes of aging, particularly in Western
countries, have changed dramatically. A child born in England in the
1780s could expect to live to thirty-five and then die of pneumonia, tu-
berculosis, diarrhea, or enteritis, then the most common causes of
death. Life expectancy today in the United States is approximately 77
years. But there is a big discrepancy between males and females: 73.6
years for men and 79.4 years for women. Death usually occurs from

heart disease, cancer, or stroke. Scientists are now asking how long a human life can be. Have we reached our maximum biological age? Because of the remarkable discoveries in molecular biology and nutrigenomics, many scientists now believe we have not.

Cynthia Kenyon, professor and director of the Hillblom Center for the Biology of Aging at the University of California in San Francisco, states, "If you understand the mechanisms of keeping things repaired, you could keep things going indefinitely." As Dr. Klatz stated recently, "We're looking at life span for the baby boomers and the generation after the baby boomers of one hundred twenty to one hundred fifty years of age." In commenting on the work in the Harvard antiaging laboratory and the relationship of xeno factors to longevity, S. Jay Olshansky, a professor of epidemiology at the University of Illinois at Chicago, asserted, "If they are right, then we will have a major weapon against everything undesirable about growing older." After considering the repair mechanisms activated by sirtuin enzymes, Toren Finkel, a cardiologist at the National Heart, Lung, and Blood Institute in Bethesda, Maryland, commented, "No one had really thought about controlling aging as a practical way to control these diseases. But it could be a powerful way of treating patients." In April 2008 David Sinclair told Barbara Walters's nationwide TV audience that the science of aging "has split the atom," and with the advent of imminent scientific discoveries, living to 120 to 150 will not be unrealistic.

Over the last hundred years, we have witnessed dramatic improvements in nutrition, housing, medical care, public health facilities, accident prevention, and infection control. The diseases that once caused early death now are uncommon. Aging itself is now considered by many to be the primary disease process. As with all disease, intense research is under way to elucidate the basic causes of aging. We have discussed several of these in earlier chapters. They include damage by free-radical reactions, suppression of the immune system with age, molecular changes between sugars and proteins that lead to a steady stiffening of tissues, and, finally, the accumulation of genetic mutations that damage mitochondria and nuclear DNA.

In a recent paper in the journal *Nature,* scientists from the department of genetics at the Erasmus Medical Center in Rotterdam, Netherlands, and also from the University of Pittsburgh tried to reconcile two conflicting hypotheses about why we age. The first is that our life span and how well we age are determined by the genes inherited from our parents. The second is that life span and fitness in old age are determined by how much damage our bodies incur over our lifetime. In their study of the metabolic pathways of progeria—a disease of premature aging—these scientists found both hypotheses to be correct. "Damage, including DNA damage, drives the functional decline we all experience as we age," they wrote. "But how we respond to that damage is determined genetically, in particular by genes that regulate the growth hormone and insulin pathways." They further stated, "This provides strong evidence that failure to repair DNA damage promotes aging—a finding that was not entirely unexpected, since DNA damage was already known to cause cancer." This shows how important it is to repair the damage that is constantly inflicted upon our genes by environmental toxins in our air, food, and water, and the deficiency of antioxidants in our body.

It is crucial that we understand the role of genes in aging and longevity: two different processes. Genes govern the cellular repair of damaged cells and regulate new cell growth, and so they indirectly determine longevity. In other words, if we lose our ability to repair damaged cells, aging occurs prematurely. If through diet, exercise, and reduced internal and external stress, our genes maintain healthy repair mechanisms, longevity ensues. It is in this context that the sirtuin gene activators found in stressed plant polyphenol molecules work. They help to repair genes and make them more resistant to damage, thereby increasing longevity by reducing cell death. With the discovery of the so-called longevity genes, which are really "super repair genes," gerontologist Richard Miller of the University of Michigan stated, "For the first time, it is abundantly clear that aging in mammals can be slowed down. If we can produce drugs that can slow down aging to the same extent we can slow aging in mice or rats, the average person would live to one hundred ten or one hundred fifteen."

The seminal observation by Clive McKay in the 1930s that calorie restriction boosts longevity by 40 percent forms the foundation for most present work on extending the life span. Roy Walford's experience in Biosphere 2 and his subsequent recommendation of the benefits of calorie restriction were another milestone. The most recent work of Joseph Baur, David Sinclair, and others demonstrating that plant-based molecules slow aging, reduce the consequences of obesity, and enhance strength and endurance opens up incredible new opportunities in preventing aging and enhancing longevity. These plant-based compounds seem to trick the body into mounting a response similar to calorie restriction but *without* calorie restriction. They are a metabolic shortcut to reducing the consequences and diseases of aging.

The amazing health benefits of calorie restriction and certain plant polyphenols are summarized in figure 11.

So, has science finally found a cure for aging? Can the many thousands of experiments in cell cultures and in animals be extrapolated to

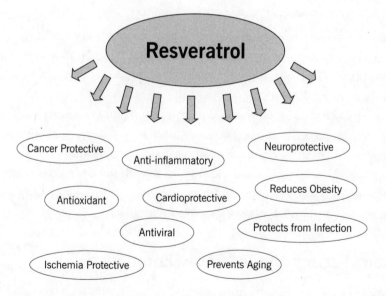

FIGURE 11 Scientific studies have demonstrated these and other health benefits of resveratrol in numerous experiential studies.

human beings? Although the study of aging is incredibly complex, there is a uniformity to our genetic pattern that crosses all life-forms. Ninety-nine percent of our genetic heritage dates back to a time before the actual appearance of humankind. In fact, only 1 percent of our genetic makeup has changed since we separated from the great ape lines more than seven million years ago. Our genetic makeup—and what activates or suppresses our genes—has changed little over millions of years. Evolution has conserved the same scarcity and longevity genes and made them standard operating equipment for virtually all species, including our own.

The sirtuin activating compounds (STACs) found in red wine grapes increase the life span of yeast by 60 percent, worms and flies by nearly 30 percent, fish by 60 percent, and mice by 25 percent. It is no surprise, therefore, that these compounds appear to have great potential benefits for humans. The question that immediately comes to mind is, What can I do to activate my own genes to enhance longevity? In humans, it will take a generation to confirm the answer. But Richard Weindruch, professor of medicine at the University of Wisconsin, has looked at the calorie restriction side of this equation for the last twenty years in monkeys. So far, 80 percent of the monkeys are still alive, and those on the restricted diet are healthier. Roughly twice as many of the monkeys in the control group have died from age-related diseases, and, perhaps most dramatically, none of the animals on the restricted diet has developed diabetes, the leading cause of death in rhesus monkeys.

Sirtuin gene and enzyme activation is the common antiaging process for both calorie restriction and sirtuin activating compounds found in stressed plants. Calorie restriction with the addition of a Xeno Diet (see chapter 19), exercise, and supplements containing STACs may be our best bet now for living longer and healthier.

Xeno Factors and Increased Endurance

From couch potatoes to professional athletes, from teenagers to the elderly, everyone would welcome a simple way to reduce muscle fatigue, increase endurance, and even eat a high-fat, high-calorie diet yet not gain weight. Two scientists at the Institute of Genetics and Molecular and Cellular Biology in France, Marie Lagouge and Johan Auwerx, have been studying the work of Guarente, Sinclair, and others who discovered the sirtuin genes. They've wondered whether resveratrol—the molecule extracted from stressed red grape skins—might also increase the number of energy-producing mitochondria and improve tissue repair following exercise.

For fifteen weeks, they gave one group of mice a daily dose of 200 milligrams per kilogram of body weight and a second group 400 milligrams per kilogram of body weight of resveratrol administered with either a regular diet or a high-fat diet. A control group was given the same diet, but without resveratrol. The results were astounding. This xeno factor dramatically increased the number of energy-producing mitochondria in muscle cells and converted type II, or fast-twitch, muscle cells (common in sprinters) to type I, or slow-twitch, muscle cells (found in endurance athletes). The treated animals were able to run literally twice as long as an untreated group, thanks to their newly increased aerobic capacity and endurance, and the higher-dose group did proportionally better than the lower-dose group. They both showed enhanced muscle strength and reduced muscle fatigue, along with improved coordination. Dr. Auwerx commented in an interview, "Resveratrol makes you look like a trained athlete without the training." He and his colleagues theorized that the same mechanism is probably at work in humans.

Most important, additional animal studies showed no evidence of toxicity in the liver or other organs from either the high fat intake or the xeno factor resveratrol. It appeared that this polyphenol molecule was able to enter the cell nucleus, activate the sirtuin enzymes, and switch the genes on or off to preserve and improve the strength and health of the tested animals, without any negative effects.

In 2007 James Smoliga, PhD, an exercise physiologist at Bloomsburg University in Pennsylvania, performed the first human trials on endurance using the Australian extract, quercetin, and resveratrol. He studied ninety sedentary subjects, divided into three groups of thirty each. The first group was given a high dose of the three plant-derived substances, and the second group was given a low dose. The third group, the control group, was given a capsule with no active ingredients. After three months, Smoglia found statistically significant increases in endurance, memory, and reaction time in the treated groups. His scientific observations, which were presented at the American College of Sports Medicine national meeting in Indianapolis in May 2008, support the potential value of using sirtuin activating compounds to enhance endurance and memory.

Currently under way is a study evaluating elite athletes, to determine if these same natural compounds may enhance endurance and strength under competitive conditions. Is it possible that compounds found in nature could replace the illicit use of steroids, growth hormone, blood doping, and other substances used to get the edge in sports competition? We should know before long.

Xeno Factors Enhance Memory

Much the same way that we lose strength, endurance, and elasticity in our muscles as we age, we also see a gradual decline in memory, reaction time, and processing of information. Approximately 1 in 3 people over fifty will experience mild cognitive impairment (MCI), which includes "slower thinking" and learning disability, along with associated memory impairment. People with MCI develop Alzheimer's disease at a rate of 10 to 15 percent per year, compared with healthy elderly individuals, who develop Alzheimer's at a rate of 1 to 2 percent per year. In the general population, the incidence of Alzheimer's doubles approximately every five years after age sixty-five, and an astounding 25 to 50 percent of people eighty-five or older will be afflicted.

Although not as obvious as sagging skin and muscles, the effects of aging on the brain can be devastating. Anything we can do to enhance cognitive function would be worthwhile. Animal studies to determine ways to slow memory loss or even improve memory are essential first steps. To learn how memory is measured in a mouse, I visited Dr. Sinclair at his Harvard laboratory. He escorted me to the pristine animal quarters, where I had to put on a dust-free white space-age garment with a surgical cap, mask, and boots. Prior to entering the animal quarters, I had to pass through a glass-enclosed chamber where powerful air jets removed any clinging dust or bacteria. Inside was a series of locked rooms with rows of mice in cages. Some mice were involved in the study of various types of cancer. One group was being evaluated for neurological impairment, including memory loss.

When I asked Sinclair, "How do you evaluate memory in a mouse?" he explained that one way is to put mice in a swimming pool where their legs aren't long enough to reach the bottom. A small platform located midway between the pool's center and one side allows the mouse to stand safely. After ninety seconds in the water, if the mouse has not found the platform, it is rescued. Then it is allowed to explore the pool again until it finds the platform. Each time it is put back in the water, it finds the platform faster. A computer tracks precisely how long it takes to find the platform each time. Using this and other assessment tools such as mazes, in 2005 scientists M. Sharma and Y. K. Gupta, from the All India Institute of Medical Sciences in New Delhi, discovered that animals engineered and grown to have Alzheimer's-like impairment had improved memory and cognitive function when given the xeno factor resveratrol.

Similar strategies can be used to assess memory in fish. They can be taught to avoid a certain stimulus (in this case, a red light in the tank) by receiving a negative stimulus when they fail to do so. When the researchers tested old fish that had been given resveratrol versus a control group without any xeno factors, they found that the age-dependent decrease in cognitive ability had been stopped: the older fish on the xeno factor maintained their processing ability as if they were still young.

In addition to Smoliga's endurance tests in sedentary people, he also performed the first study using the Australian extract, resveratrol, and quercetin to assess memory and reaction time. He used a computer software test called ImPACT (Immediate Post-Concussion Assessment and Cognitive Testing), which I developed with Mark Lovell, PhD, to determine the degree of memory impairment and loss of reaction time following a cerebral concussion in athletes. It is the standard of care in the National Football League, the National Hockey League, NASCAR, World Wrestling Entertainment, and more than two thousand high schools and colleges in the United States. It is the most validated and reliable test for memory and reaction time in sports today. Using ImPACT, Smoliga found an improvement in visual and verbal memory and in reaction time that could be measured to 1/100th of a second in the treated group. It appears that this is one of the few nutraceutical agents shown to enhance memory and reaction time in normal, healthy, sedentary individuals. Further confirmatory tests on larger samples of subjects are needed.

Chapters 10 through 17 examine in depth resveratrol's possible role in treating and even preventing common health problems such as cardio-vascular disease, diabetes, cancer, stroke, degenerative brain diseases, excess weight, and inflammatory conditions.

Chapter 10

Diabetes

*I think a lot of people were also inhibited by previous failures.
. . . To overlook those things and still go ahead with the hope,
almost with the expectation, of success was essential.*

—DR. C. H. BEST, THE CODISCOVERER OF INSULIN

*The thing always happens that you believe in; and the belief
in a thing makes it happen.*

—FRANK LLOYD WRIGHT

Diabetes costs our nation more than the conflicts in Iraq, Afghanistan, and the global war on terrorism combined—an estimated $174 billion per year. With over 60 percent of Americans overweight or obese, one million new cases are added a year. If current trends continue, 1 in 3 people born in 2000 and 1 in 2 members of minorities will develop diabetes in their lifetime. The personal cost from its associated blindness, kidney failure, heart attacks, strokes, poor wound healing, infections, blood sugar complications, and amputated limbs is inestimable.

Diabetes is a disease of sugar and fat metabolism caused by problems with insulin secretion by the pancreas, or with the insulin sensitivity of the cells. Insulin, a hormone, facilitates the uptake of sugar required by every cell to produce energy. There are two primary types of diabetes. Type 1, which is the more serious, develops when the body's immune system destroys the insulin-secreting cells in the pancreas. This type accounts for 5 to 10 percent of all cases and usually strikes children and young adults, although it can occur at any age. Type 2 diabetes, often called "adult-onset diabetes," accounts for 90 to 95 percent of all diagnosed cases. This type usually begins when cells do not use insulin properly and develop resistance to it. To compensate, the pancreas attempts to produce more insulin and gradually loses the ability to do so, or burns out.

Type 2 diabetes is associated with advanced age, obesity, a family history of diabetes, physical inactivity, and ethnicity. African Americans, Hispanic/Latino Americans, Native Americans, some Asian Americans, and Native Hawaiian or Pacific Islanders are at particularly high risk of type 2 diabetes. Both types can lead to organ damage and complications such as blindness, heart and kidney failure, strokes, and infections, through three main mechanisms: glycation (sugar molecules attaching themselves to fat and protein), free radicals/oxidative stress, and inflammation.

Today approximately twenty-one million Americans, or 7 percent of the population, suffer from diabetes. One in four has the disease or is at risk of getting it. Six million are unaware they have it. Overeating, starchy diets, and lack of exercise are the primary causes. Foods that contain a significant amount of carbohydrates—grains, fruits, vegetables, and beans—are rated on a scale according to how high they raise blood sugar levels, called the "glycemic index," or GI (see table 3). A recent analysis of the dietary habits of nearly two million healthy men and women showed that people who ate the diets highest in foods that spike blood sugar levels (high-GI foods) were more likely to develop not only diabetes but also heart disease, gallstones, and some types of cancer. According to Alan Barclay of the University of Sydney in Australia, lead author of the study, "If you have constantly high blood sugar and insulin levels due to a high-GI diet, you may literally wear out your pancreas over time. Eventually it may lead to diabetes."

Medical anthropologists refer to diabetes and obesity as "diseases of civilization." It was when aboriginal populations began to adopt a high-sugar, high-fat, "Western" diet for the first time that obesity and diabetes suddenly appeared. The Pima Indians of Arizona and the indigenous people of Hawaii provide dramatic demonstrations of this phenomenon. In both instances, the abandonment of their traditional plant-rich, high-fiber diet was followed by skyrocketing rates of diabetes, obesity, and cancer.

Glycemic Index and Glycemic Load

The glycemic index was developed to help researchers understand the spikes and troughs of blood sugar. This index ranks food according to its ability to release sugar into the bloodstream. A food with a high glycemic index (GI), like potatoes, white bread, or cornflakes, raises blood sugar and insulin levels more quickly than one with a low GI, like green peas or carrots. Another index is the glycemic load (GL): the number of grams of carbohydrate in the food multiplied by its GI. The GL provides a better indicator of the amount of insulin needed to digest a given food. The amount needed is based on the quantity of carbohydrates and how fast they are converted to glucose. For example, carrots have a GI of 47, and pasta, 44. But because pasta is so high in carbohydrates, it has a GL of 21 versus 4 for carrots. High-GL diets are strongly associated with diabetes (see table 3).

Americans are eating and drinking themselves to death. Studies indicate that a reduction in the intake of refined sugar and a thirty-

TABLE 3

Classification	GI Range	Example
Low GI	55 or less	Most fruits and vegetables (except potatoes, watermelon, and sweet corn), whole grains, pasta, beans, and lentils
Medium GI	56 to 69	Brown rice, croissant, basmati rice, and sucrose
High GI	70 or more	Cornflakes, baked potato, white rice, white bread, candy bars, sodas, sports drinks

minute walk a day would cut the incidence of diabetes in the United States by around half. But just the opposite is occurring, as Americans consume more sugar products and become more sedentary. As a result, diabetes has been compared to a sleeping giant that is ready to awaken and overwhelm our current health care system. In the last twenty-five years, the number of adults between the ages of eighteen and seventy-nine with newly diagnosed diabetes almost tripled, from approximately 493,000 to 1.4 million. By the year 2025, it is predicted that around 9 percent of the U.S. population will have diabetes, or approximately twenty-five million to thirty million people.

What does all this have to do with xeno factors? To answer that, let's take a look at the current drugs used to treat diabetes and then see how xeno factors may play a part.

In type 1 diabetes, injections of insulin (see box) keep the body's level of blood sugar under control. In type 2 diabetes, where cells still produce insulin, but not enough, oral medications are the first line of treatment. These drugs lower blood sugar by increasing insulin output from the "tired" pancreas and by improving insulin sensitivity. Most scientists believe that lower blood sugar will decrease the complications of diabetes, including heart attacks, blindness, and kidney failure.

To this end, nine classes of oral drugs—five approved in the past decade—are available for type 2 diabetes. But relatively little is known about their risks. As Dr. Victor Montori, a Mayo Clinic diabetes authority, put it, "My patients can't choose medications on the basis of benefit. They only chose the least painful poison." Reported side effects include weight gain, nausea, liver toxicity, visual impairment, and increased fracture risk in women.

In fact, in June 2007 Dr. Steven Nissen, chair of cardiovascular medicine at the Cleveland Clinic, and his colleagues made international headlines when the *New England Journal of Medicine* published their findings on the complications of heart failure from the widely used diabetes drugs Avandia and Actos. Nissen and his team found that patients on Avandia had a 43 percent higher risk of heart attack. The U.S. Food and Drug Administration (FDA) subsequently

Discovery of Insulin

Prior to 1921, a diagnosis of diabetes was an automatic death sentence. In 1920 a Canadian surgeon named Frederick Banting had an inspiration. He knew there was a connection between the pancreas and diabetes, and guessed that the pancreas's digestive juice was destroying the cells that made whatever substance the pancreas produced to regulate the level of sugar in the blood. Dr. Banting thought that if he could stop the pancreas from working but keep the cells going that produced this substance, he should be able to isolate the stuff. John Macleod, the head of the department of physiology at the University of Toronto, initially scoffed at Banting's idea, but he acceded to the pleadings of his assistant, Dr. Charles Best, and allowed Banting to perform experiments on ten diabetic dogs. Macleod then left for a holiday in his native Scotland in May 1921.

By August Banting and his team had extracted from cells in the pancreas a substance they called insulin (from the Latin for island or islets). They administered this substance to diabetic dogs with abnormally high blood sugar and became ecstatic when they saw the animals' blood sugar decrease dramatically. Back from his holiday and still skeptical, Macleod had them repeat the experiments—with the same findings. Within six weeks, the researchers had purified the substance, then boldly gave it to a human for the first time: a fourteen-year-old boy dying of diabetes, who would become the first of millions to be saved from this dreaded disease. While not a cure, insulin continues to save millions of lives worldwide. In 1923 the Nobel Prize was awarded to Banting and Macleod for their discovery.

asked the makers of Avandia and Actos to add a warning to their packaging about the risks of congestive heart failure.

This revelation of unintended but potentially fatal complications from drugs that help in one area but harm in another is similar to the Vioxx and Bextra fiasco. Touted as the optimal anti-inflammatory drugs for arthritis, these COX-2 inhibitors were removed from the market five years after their introduction, owing to an increase in fatal heart attacks, not to mention the cost in human life as well as the loss of billions of dollars of revenue and countless lawsuits against the manufacturers.

Since the therapeutic effects of all current drugs used to treat type 2 diabetes depend either directly or indirectly on insulin, the development of a new class of insulin-independent drugs that lower blood sugar would be tremendously valuable. Among the earliest scientists to investigate the effects of naturally occurring polyphenols on insulin secretion were C. S. Hii and his associate S. L. Howell, from the University of Adelaide in Australia. In 1985 they discovered that two components in red wine and grape juice, quercetin and *epicatechin,* enhanced insulin release in rats by 44 percent to 70 percent in certain cells. After their report, the therapeutic use of those natural compounds for diabetes lay dormant in the medical literature until quite recently.

In 2003 Dr. Mahmood Vessal and his colleagues in the department of biochemistry at Shiraz University in Iran administered quercetin to a group of diabetic rats and discovered that it regenerated pancreatic cells and increased insulin release. In 2004 Najim Al-Awwadi and his fellow researchers from the University of Montpellier in France confirmed that quercetin reduced blood sugar and decreased appetite in diabetic and healthy animals.

The development of type 2 diabetes is related to increased amounts of fat circulating in the bloodstream. In 2005 scientist Edward Park, working at Brock University in Canada, discovered that resveratrol appears to counter the effects of elevated free fatty acids, allowing normal insulin uptake in muscle cells. Danna Breen from the same university reported on the amazing action of resveratrol. She found that this polyphenol could increase glucose absorption in a manner different from insulin and was not dependent on the action of enzymes typically needed to allow glucose to enter the cell.

In January 2006 Hui-Chen Su and his associates in Taiwan evaluated the effect of resveratrol in diabetic rats. They confirmed the findings of previous investigators, and showed that resveratrol stimulated the uptake of glucose by liver, fat, and muscle cells. Again, resveratrol appeared to act through a mechanism different from that of insulin.

These observations on resveratrol and the mechanisms of glucose, insulin, and fat metabolism—which are supported by the work of David Sinclair and Joe Baur, as well as by the work of Marie Lagouge and Johan Auwerx in France—are so revolutionary that a pharmaceutical company called Sirtris was formed with the specific goal of developing resveratrol-like compounds to give people the same boosts in blood sugar control that resveratrol gave mice. After quickly raising $165 million, Sirtris analyzed nearly five hundred thousand compounds and has targeted diabetes as the first disease to treat. The company is presently evaluating its resveratrol product in diabetic patients. Preliminary results indicate that the resveratrol-like compound is safe, increases insulin sensitivity, enhances blood sugar control, and has huge potential to safely help millions of people.

Quercetin, also found in red wine and red grape juice, has likewise shown promise in animals with diabetes. It appears to be effective in reducing the high spike in insulin that occurs when sugary food is ingested; sensing the sugar, the pancreas releases this jolt of insulin to help drive it into cells. These insulin peaks are responsible for the hunger cravings that occur soon after someone eats a meal loaded with processed sugar.

In addition to reducing these insulin peaks and slowing the absorption of sugars, quercetin is also a potent inhibitor of sugars in the intestine, contributing to a steadier energy state. In a 2005 Chilean study, investigators confirmed that not only quercetin but several other plant polyphenols found in grape skins (like *myricetin* and catechin gallate) also slowed sugar absorption in the intestines. All of these naturally derived xeno factors—resveratrol, quercetin, myricetin, catechins, and more—hold great potential for diabetic management in the near term.

One of the most dreaded complications of diabetes is diabetic neuropathy, in which the blood vessels that supply blood to nerves may be blocked, literally causing "strokes" to these nerves. This results in constant, intense, burning pain, usually in the legs but also in the arms. No medication is known to fully relieve it. In 2006 investigators at Panjab University in India evaluated the ability of resveratrol to reduce diabetic neuropathic pain. Looking at various inflammatory markers associated with this pain, they discovered that daily oral intake of resveratrol at 5, 10, and 20 milligrams per kilogram of body weight significantly reduced pain sensitivity in treated animals with induced nerve damage. For an average male weighing 70 kilograms, that would amount to 350 to 1,400 mg a day, a reasonable dose.

What, then, is the relationship between xeno factors and diabetes? Through their action of decreasing insulin resistance, enhancing glucose's ability to enter the cells, and stabilizing weight, polyphenols provide a complementary way to attack the disease. Additionally, studies have confirmed that polyphenols are potent anti-inflammatories, that they reduce free radicals, and that they inhibit the formation of damaging advanced glycation end products, or AGEs.

It is the prevention of diabetic complications that may be the greater role for plant-produced polyphenols. As discussed earlier in theories of aging, these glycation end products (AGEs) are formed by a cellular interaction of blood proteins that become bound to circulating glucose molecules. And the AGEs can occur more frequently in poorly controlled diabetics. These AGEs can stick to blood vessel walls and induce the development of diabetic vascular complications.

We are just beginning to understand how these naturally occurring compounds ingested over thousands of years activate ancient genetic pathways to enhance health and prolong longevity. But one of the most exciting possibilities is their potential for drug-free management of the diabetes pandemic.

Chapter 11

Cardio Protection

Knowing is not enough—we must apply. Willing is not enough—we must do.

—GOETHE

"Stat page, stat page—Dr. Maroon to the emergency room." I was in the operating room, just completing the microsurgical removal of an egg-size brain tumor, when the page crackled over the PA system. I wasn't on call for trauma, so I had no idea what was going on. I jogged down the back stairs, taking a shortcut from the operating room to the ER, and as I passed the triage nurse sitting at her desk, she looked up and said, "Bed 16, Dr. Maroon." There on the gurney, covered by a white sheet and clutching his chest in pain, was an anxious, pale, sweaty fifty-one-year-old male—my father.

"Dad! What happened?"

Wincing in pain, he said, "I had just finished a large lunch and was walking up the stairs to the bedroom for a little nap when the chest pain hit me, like someone just sat on my chest. Your mother called the ambulance, and here I am."

My father grew up during the Great Depression and lived through the Second World War, so he knew firsthand about adversity and the toughness it takes to survive. Although he was a competitive boxer in his youth, by the time he was thirty-five, with a family of three and a vending machine route that was expanding, my father was no longer physically active. A "healthy" steak, now that he could afford it, became the mainstay of his diet. As a medical student, I diagnosed his hypertension when he was forty-five. I learned more about heart disease, which made me more conscious of his lifestyle and his major cardiac risk factors: rich foods, no exercise, hypertension, and an apple-shaped, moderately obese body. My warnings to him became so frequent that he finally said, "You're not *my* father. If you continue to badger me about how I should lead my life, I don't want to see you anymore." I got the message and consoled myself that at least he didn't smoke, drink, or have diabetes.

Four years later, here we were. The coronary catheter lab told us that all the major vessels of his heart were lined with hard plaque deposits, and when the cardiac surgeons reviewed his angiogram, they declined to operate. "The chances that he'll die in surgery are too high," they said. For the next five years, my father took his blood pressure medicine, lost weight, modified his diet, and continued to expand his business. Then the old habits returned, along with the weight, the hypertension, and the shortness of breath.

Finally, on a terribly cold February morning, while still working at his office at one in the morning, my father suffered a massive fatal heart attack. The autopsy confirmed that his heart had actually ruptured from the weakness caused by blocked arteries and lack of blood supply.

What is the point of this story? I want to describe my firsthand experience with the number one killer in the United States. After sharing my own example of everything not to do to avoid a heart attack, now I would like to explore what causes heart attacks, the best ways to prevent them, and how natural approaches—in particular the use of polyphenols such as resveratrol, quercetin, and other compounds found in red grape skins—may provide valuable new protection for the heart, along with diet and exercise.

What Is a Heart Attack?

As people's life spans have increased and our diet has moved away from what we ate thousands of years ago as hunter-gatherers, heart

disease has increased, but it was not until 1912 that we began to understand the mechanisms involved. That year Professor James Herrick, a
physician at the University of Chicago, published his landmark paper
"Clinical Features of Sudden Obstruction of the Coronary Arteries." In
it he correlated autopsy findings of blocked arteries in the heart with
patients who had also complained of chest pain over several months or
years and then died suddenly. Dr. Hemick coined the term "heart attack," or *myocardial infarction,* to describe what occurs when a part
of the heart muscle dies or is damaged due to an inadequate supply of
oxygen-rich blood to that area.

Dr. Friedrich Hoffmann, the chief professor in medicine at the University of Halle in Germany in the early 1700s, stated, "The origins of
coronary heart disease lie in the reduced passage of blood within the
coronary arteries." He used the term *atherosclerosis,* from *athero*
(meaning "paste") and *sclerosis* ("hardness"), to describe coronary arteries filled with calcium, blood clots, and cellular debris that blocked
the coronary arteries to produce heart disease.

Until quite recently, scientists accepted the idea that a heart attack
was caused primarily by a plumbing problem, much the way that mineral deposits and rust build up inside water pipes over time. The
human heart beats roughly one hundred thousand times per day, cy-
cling six quarts of blood through the sixty thousand miles of blood vessels in our bodies. It stood to reason that deposits would accumulate
in this elaborate system and eventually cause blockages, leading to a
heart attack.

The New Theory of Heart Disease

Coronary artery disease, or hardening of the coronary arteries, is indeed the cause of most heart attacks. The problem is that as much as
half the time, sudden death is the first symptom of heart disease. It was
well established that elevated cholesterol levels, high blood pressure,
diabetes, tobacco use, obesity, and sedentary lifestyles were all major
risk factors associated with progressive artery blockage, but they
showed up in only half of all fatal heart attacks. So what caused the rest?

In the early 1990s, scientists began to look beyond the composition of the clots blocking blood vessels to the lining of the vessels themselves, called the *endothelium*. Its functions include regulating inflammation and immune reactions, the tone of blood vessels (their ability to contract and widen, or dilate), clotting, the formation of new blood vessels, and so on. Like the skin on the outer surface of the body, the endothelium is subject to a multitude of disease processes as it performs its vital regulatory functions. So important is the study of the endothelium that this research has become the basis of a new frontier called *endotheliology*. As scientists struggle to find ways to avert heart attacks, which kill more than seven million people worldwide each year, the endothelium seems to lie at the heart of the problem.

Many components circulating in the blood can damage the arteries' inner lining. These include glucose (sugar), trans-fatty acids, low-density lipoproteins (LDLs), free radicals, and *cytokines*—signaling molecules that can turn inflammation on and off. To prevent heart disease and understand the role of xeno factors in prevention, we need to understand the five stages leading to a heart attack. These are: (1) the accumulation and oxidation of fat by free radicals; (2) inflammation within the blood vessel itself; (3) a markedly decreased vascular tone and decreased elasticity of the blood vessels; (4) increased clotting that results in coronary thrombosis, or the sudden obstruction of the coronary arteries, as described by Herrick; and (5) the damage or death of the heart muscle itself (see figure 12).

Let's take a close look at the remarkable promise that xeno factors offer by fighting heart disease at each of these five stages.

Xeno Factors and Cardio Protection

Heart disease, cancer, Alzheimer's disease, and many forms of arthritis all have one common link to our age-old immunological defense mechanism: inflammation. Inflammation is the body's first defense against infection and trauma. Now scientists have finally connected the dots, giving researchers renewed hopes that a remedy for inflammation could possibly prevent the many major diseases that ail us.

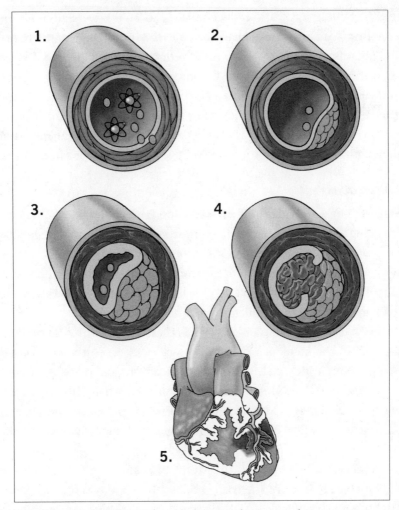

FIGURE 12 The five stages leading to a heart attack.

In the search for this holy grail, drug companies are spending billions of dollars on researching new drugs and are exploring new ways to use existing drugs. Celebrex, a so-called COX-2 inhibitor used primarily for arthritis because of its anti-inflammatory effects, is being evaluated to see if it can prevent breast cancer, slow memory loss in Alzheimer's disease, and eliminate polyp development in the intestines. Statin drugs, thought to reduce the incidence of heart attacks by reducing cholesterol, also reduce inflammation; this reduction may be their primary cardio-protective mechanism. Aspirin, the grandfather of anti-inflammatory drugs, known for reducing the incidence of heart attacks, is also being tested on colon cancer and Alzheimer's disease. And very recently, natural substances high in xeno factors—resveratrol, quercetin, catechin, and the other polyphenol compounds—have shown remarkable early signs of effectiveness against inflammation. But their anti-inflammatory properties are just part of their promise.

The Process

Stage 1: The Antioxidant Effect: Reducing Free Radicals

Diets high in fat, particularly from meat and hydrogenated vegetable oils, or so-called trans-fatty acids, found abundantly in French fries, some cakes, and margarine, are extremely damaging to the endothelium. In fact, trans fats appear to increase the risk of heart disease more than any other food product, even at very low levels. A 2 percent increase in calories from trans-fatty acids is associated with a 23 percent increase in the incidence of coronary artery disease. It is no wonder that the New York City Department of Health required 20,000 restaurants and 14,000 food suppliers to eliminate partially hydrogenated oils from their food. Other states are following suit, and Denmark and Canada are actually considering legislation to eliminate all industrially produced trans-fatty acids from their food supply.

After being processed by the liver, fats accumulate in the blood in the form of cholesterol and triglycerides. There are two primary types of cholesterol molecules: LDL, or "bad" low-density lipoprotein; and HDL, or "good" high-density lipoprotein, which has been referred to as the "arterial wall garbage barge" because of its ability to haul away bad cholesterol from clogged arteries.

If the balance tips toward LDL and other toxic food by-products, the endothelium becomes irritated and causes microscopic cracks to develop in the lining of the blood vessel. These cracks release free radicals that oxidize or degrade the LDL. The accumulation of free radicals in oxidized LDL leads to the next stage of coronary disease.

When an oxygen molecule is added to LDL cholesterol, this creates a fatty substance that can attack the membranes of surrounding cells, particularly the endothelium. This deterioration of membrane lipids (fats), known as lipid peroxidation, is extremely destructive to the blood vessel lining. Our bodies use antioxidants in our diet to counter these destructive effects. In 1995 Dr. M. I. Furman at the University of Massachusetts Medical Center evaluated the effects of red wine on LDL. He found that the people in the treatment group, who drank one and a half glasses of red wine per day, lowered their level of lipid peroxide (the toxic material) by an average of 40 percent.

In 1998 S. V. Nigdikar and associates at Papworth Hospital in Cambridge, England, took this one step further, demonstrating that an alcohol-free powder of a red wine polyphenol extract had similar antioxidant effects, both in the blood and in LDL cholesterol. This confirmed that although alcohol in red wine may contribute to cardio protection, the main antioxidant protection comes from polyphenols.

There are several mechanisms for this protection. As free-radical scavengers, these xeno factors prevent free radicals from "stealing" electrons from the membranes of normal cells, and this action in turn prevents any destructive effect. Other studies have shown that polyphenols bind to LDL cholesterol, thus protecting it from peroxidation. The bottom line is that the polyphenols found in xeno factors significantly inhibit or prevent the first stage in the development of a heart attack through their antioxidant effect.

Stage 2: The Anti-inflammatory Xeno Effect
When oxidized LDL and fat just under the endothelium accumulate, they attract white blood cells circulating in the bloodstream. These white cells, called macrophages, proceed to ingest the cholesterol in an attempt to remove it. The now fat-laden microphages (known as "foam cells" because they appear plump and white under the microscope) create a significant inflammatory reaction. Smooth muscle cells form a cap over the injury site in the blood vessel lining; calcium accumulates here and forms a material similar to bone—hence the term

hardening of the arteries. The word *plaque* refers to this combination of foam cells, smooth muscle cells, and lipid accumulation, which has a cheesy appearance.

The discovery of *nuclear factor kappa B* (*NF-κB*) is critical in the understanding of inflammation (see figures 13 and 14). The NF-κB molecule is a protein that acts as a switch to turn inflammation on and

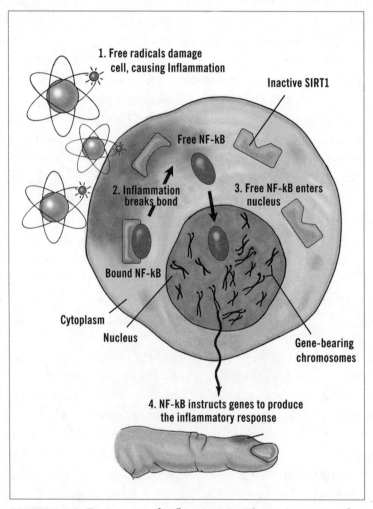

FIGURE 13 Four steps of inflammation: The transcription factor NF-κB perpetuates the inflammatory response.

off in the body. Known as the body's "smoke detector," it can detect substances such as infectious agents, free radicals, and other bad actors. In response, it turns on particular genes that promote production of inflammatory cytokines that in turn try to kill or isolate the invading agent through the inflammatory response.

When the membranes of the surrounding cells sense the toxic debris of the plaque, NF-κB facilitates the production of chemicals that promote and maintain the normally protective inflammatory state. These agents attract defensive white blood cells to the site of inflammation and enhance cellular proliferation and growth. In the case of the coronary arteries, however, the inflammation response persists

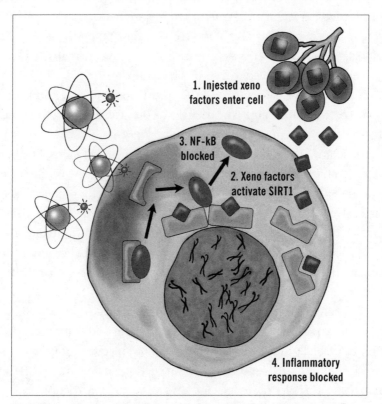

FIGURE 14 Xeno factors activating SIRT1 to block the inflammation and reduce cellular damage.

and will not stop until the muscle cells just under the endothelium grow over the site of irritation in an attempt to cover the debris.

It is through blocking or inhibiting NF-κB activity that aspirin; non-steroidal anti-inflammatories like Celebrex, Aleve, and ibuprofen; and natural compounds like white willow bark work to block inflammation. Multiple lines of laboratory studies indicate that xeno factors such as resveratrol, quercetin, and others act as potent anti-inflammatory agents through a similar action on NF-κB.

Stage 3: The Vascular Dilation Effect
(or the Viagra Connection)

The coronary arteries widen and constrict to vary blood supply to the heart muscle under different circumstances. When we walk up a steep hill or exercise vigorously, our blood vessels automatically dilate to bring more oxygen-carrying blood to the heart. When the physical activity is over, the blood vessels return to a more normal size. Artery walls encrusted with plaque lose this flexibility.

A substance called *nitric oxide,* produced by the endothelium, promotes relaxation and constriction of the arterial smooth muscle. This bit of biochemistry led to the discovery in 1996 of one of the largest-selling drugs ever: Viagra. One of the earliest signs of athero-sclerotic changes, or hardening of the arteries, is the inability of the endothelium to make nitric oxide, which would allow the arteries to dilate. Because of the general protective effects of polyphenols, scientists set out to determine if these compounds might enhance nitric oxide production. Indeed, it has been confirmed that resveratrol enhances the production of nitric oxide, allowing arteries to dilate in times of need.

The xeno factors also block a substance called *endothelin-1 (ET-1)*, which is a potent constrictor of blood vessels and also stimulates smooth vascular muscle cells to cover up the plaque within the blood vessel. Inhibiting ET-1 production, protecting against atherosclerotic changes in the blood vessel, blocking vascular constriction, and en-hancing vascular enlargement are all ways in which natural xeno factors work to provide cardio protection at this third stage of cardiac disease development.

Stage 4: The Xeno Factor and Blood Clotting

As material continues to build up inside the blood vessel, it can accumulate to the point where blood flow is markedly reduced and then finally blocked. More commonly, however, the arterial plaque can break up, exposing the underlying cellular debris to the rapidly flowing bloodstream. The body senses this as an injury and sends *platelets,* one of the main components of blood, to the injured area to form protective clots. These sticky platelets quickly pile up. A sudden heart attack occurs when blood flow is abruptly cut off by the platelet thrombus, or clot, leading to the death of heart muscles that depend on richly oxygenated blood for survival.

In 2002 Zhenghin Wang and colleagues at Peking University in China fed rabbits a high-cholesterol diet and found that the platelets involved in clotting became stickier. When they gave another group of animals the same diet plus resveratrol, it blocked the platelet aggregation, or clumping. In an extensive review of this subject, Beata Olas and Barbara Wachowicz from the Institute of Biochemistry at the University of Lodz, Poland, listed the various mechanisms by which resveratrol affects blood platelet functions. They concluded that resveratrol unquestionably inhibits platelet function, although the mechanism is quite complex. In 2000 Italian researchers evaluating quercetin and catechin also found similar antiplatelet actions. These studies, as well as many others, concluded that one of the primary positive effects of xeno factors in protecting against cardiovascular disease involves its antiplatelet activity, which decreases the tendency of platelets to cluster and block the arteries that nourish the heart.

Stage 5: Stopping the Heart Attack

As we've seen, a heart attack occurs when a coronary artery no longer supplies blood to a particular part of the heart. Heart failure, which is often related to a heart attack, results when the heart muscle is unable to pump blood at a rate that meets the needs of the body's tissues. In essence, if the pumping action of the heart is too weak, the body can be starved of blood—and therefore oxygen. With heart failure, the heart enlarges, its chambers dilate, and the heart's life-sustaining ability to pump deteriorates.

In 2005 Dr. Jyothish Pillai and his associates at the department of molecular biology and pharmacology at the University of Chicago and Washington University School of Medicine in St. Louis were investigating the mechanism of heart failure when they found that a specific enzyme found in cardiac cells is activated by free radicals, calcium, and magnesium released by cellular injury from a heart attack. When this enzyme, *poly (ADP-ribose) polymerase-1* (or *PARP*), is overactivated, it results in heart cell death. It also suppresses the heart cell's mitochondria, or nucleic power plants, leading to an energy deficit in cells that survive.

In studying how PARP activation causes cardiac cell death, these scientists discovered a direct link to the SIRT1 enzyme: PARP reduces the activity of SIRT1. Could the same process also work in reverse, to the benefit of the heart? Dr. Pillai and his colleagues were familiar with the work of Guarente, Sinclair, and Baur. In 2006 they too studied activation of the sirtuin enzyme with resveratrol and discovered that it indeed protected the heart cells against PARP-mediated cell death. SIRT1 activation helped preserve cell function.

Other scientists went a step further to see if resveratrol could serve a cardio-protective role if taken *before* a heart attack. In 2006 Karel Bezstarosti and his associates from the Erasmus Medical Center in the Netherlands reported the remarkable result that animals pretreated with resveratrol and then subjected to heart attacks showed a decreased myocardial death rate compared with animals not administered resveratrol.

A study by C. H. R. Wallace at the department of pharmacology at the University of Alberta in Canada evaluated the ability of a red wine extract to decrease the electrical irritability of a heart muscle cell. This would be useful in cases of cardiac rhythm disturbances, which can lead to sudden cardiac death. He concluded that both resveratrol and quercetin could significantly inhibit abnormal electrical flow through a heart muscle cell.

In sum, xeno factors, natural products readily available in our food, can help protect us against heart disease at every stage in its development, and can help ameliorate its life-threatening effects when a heart attack occurs. Unfortunately, my father did not know about these xeno factors; nor do most of the one million people in the United States each year who suffer a heart attack.

Prevention is still the key to survival. The United States performs three times as many invasive heart procedures per one hundred thousand people as France, Japan, and Great Britain yet still has the highest death rate from heart disease. Contrary to popular belief, although these heart surgeries may decrease symptoms, they don't decrease heart attacks or extend life for most patients. In June 2007 Dr. Darwin Labarthe and his colleagues from the Centers for Disease Control and Prevention reported in the *New England Journal of Medicine* that preventive methods of lowering heart risk save as many lives as treatment. Quitting smoking, lowering blood pressure, and reducing other known health risks have prevented as many heart deaths over the last twenty years as have costly high-tech treatments. I believe that risk reduction plus supplementing a healthy diet with xeno factors may be the optimal preventive strategy for heart disease.

Chapter 12

The Anticancer Effect

With cancer we have two options, medically and emotionally: give up or fight like hell.

—LANCE ARMSTRONG

Karen did not expect to die at age thirty-seven from colon cancer. Two years after giving birth to her third child, she had been told by her physician that her painful abdominal cramping was mild irritable bowel syndrome, and since her upper GI X-rays were normal, no additional studies were necessary. Reassured, she enthusiastically jumped back into her life as a soccer mom, devoted wife, and Sunday school teacher. That is, until the cough she developed just wouldn't let up.

Another visit to her doctor led to a chest X-ray and then a CT scan of the lungs. Biopsies revealed the worst: cancer, most likely from the colon. An abdominal CT scan, blood tests, and a sigmoidoscopy confirmed that the primary location was the colon and that the cancer had also spread to the liver and ovaries.

After I received the call from her father, my cousin, I canceled my patient appointments and drove to his home, where Karen, her parents, and I sat around the large glass kitchen table. Then the barrage of questions began. How did this happen? Could it be cured—or treated? What about chemotherapy, radiation therapy, and their side effects? What was the best cancer center in the country? Who was the best doctor to treat it? Could this cancer have been prevented?

I learned early in my career that despite the gravest prognosis, hope must not be denied to any patient. Powerful emotions such as anxiety, fear, and depression impair the body's natural cellular defenses. I have also found that information, trust, and confidence in the physician-healer are the best ways to allay fear and enhance recommended treatment. So I began to lay out, as I had done so many times before, answers to their torrent of questions.

I began by explaining that our bodies are composed of over one hundred trillion cells, each of which is a sort of biochemical factory that produces energy, manufactures proteins, and replicates. Each cell has its own regulatory system controlled by genes on chromosomes within the nucleus of every cell. I described cancer as a disease caused by genes gone haywire—specifically those genes that regulate cell growth. There is a constant balance in every cell between so-called *oncogenes* (genes involved in uncontrolled cell growth and proliferation) and *tumor suppressor genes* (genes that turn off division and replicating mechanisms). When the balance tips in favor of the oncogenes—from environmental and genetic causes—cells escape the normal control mechanisms of the body and continue to divide and grow unchecked.

Cancer can involve any organ of the body; the most common fatal types involve the prostate gland, the breast, the lungs, and the colon—the so-called big four—but no organ or tissue is exempt. Cancer claims more than five million American lives each year and accounts for more than 12 percent of the world's mortality. Lung cancer is the leading cause of U.S. cancer deaths, followed by intestinal cancer. In the United States, cancer is the second-leading cause of death (after heart disease) and is responsible for approximately one death in every four (see table 4).

But why did this cancer occur in a thirty-seven-year-old woman who exercised, didn't smoke, and was not overweight—all factors associated with a lower incidence of colon cancer? Could it be related to her fairly typical American diet, which was somewhat high in well-cooked meat, saturated fat, and trans-fatty acids? Or to the stress and compromise of her immune system associated with her work and fam-

TABLE 4

Type of Cancer	Deaths per Year	New Cases Diagnosed per Year	Five-year Survival Rate
Lung	160,390	213,380	16%
Colon	52,180	112,340	65%
Breast	40,190	180,510	89%
Pancreas	33,370	37,170	5%
Prostate	27,050	218,890	99%

SOURCE: NATIONAL CANCER INSTITUTE.

ily? Or to some unidentified environmental factors? All are associated with increased risk of colon cancer. Or was there a genetic predisposition that had been triggered by any of the above?

I listed all of the lifestyle factors that contribute to genetic mutations and cancer, including smoking, excess drinking, lack of exercise, and diets high in processed meat, saturated fat, sugar, trans-fatty acids, and vegetable oils. (At that point, Karen's father, a two-pack-a-day smoker, stubbed out his cigarette.) Other contributors include environmental pollutants, such as impure water, electromagnetic radiation, toxic waste products, pesticides and hormones in our food, and air pollutants from industrial sources.

But what effect do these practices and agents have on cells that turns them into ruthless killers? To understand this, as well as the optimal treatment for any cancer, we need to understand how and why cancers form, grow, and then seed throughout the body. From studying thousands of experimentally induced cancers in animals, scientists have determined that tumor development consists of three separate but closely linked stages: tumor *initiation,* tumor *promotion,* and tumor *progression.*

Initiation, the first stage of cancer development, occurs when free radicals attack the membrane of the cell, the mitochondria, and the DNA in the cell's nucleus. Injury to the DNA leads to mutations and, if unchecked, to the production of a malignancy.

Top Five Cancer-Causing Foods

- Hot dogs
- Processed meats and bacon
- Doughnuts
- French fries
- Chips, crackers, cookies

These products contain: hydrogenated oils (trans fats), which, besides being a cancer factor, promote heart disease and belly fat; acrylamides, which are created during the frying process; and sodium nitrite (and nitrates), which are added to processed meats, hot dogs, bacon, and any other meat that needs a reddish color to look "fresh." During digestion, sodium nitrite is converted to nitrosamine, which is a carcinogen, or cancer-causing agent.

As we've seen, the reactive nature of free radicals, and their ability to destabilize almost every molecule they contact, makes them harmful to normal human cells. Free radicals are normal by-products of the cell's energy-producing mitochondria—much like the exhaust from burning gasoline in a combustion engine. The body has systems to remove them, but to combat the overproduction of free radicals accelerated by improper diet, environmental pollution, and the body's own normal production, the body turns to antioxidants like vitamins C, E, and beta-carotene to neutralize their destructive effects.

The second stage in the development of cancer is the promotion phase. If the first line of defense fails to prevent the initiation of cancer, cancer cells can proliferate. This is a lengthy and still reversible process in which actively dividing precancerous cells accumulate and enlarge. This phase of rapid cell division is enhanced by inflammation, not only at the site but also throughout the body. Vegetable oils such as corn and safflower oil, manmade trans-fatty acids, and saturated fats found in meat and fatty fried foods all contribute to this silent inflammation,

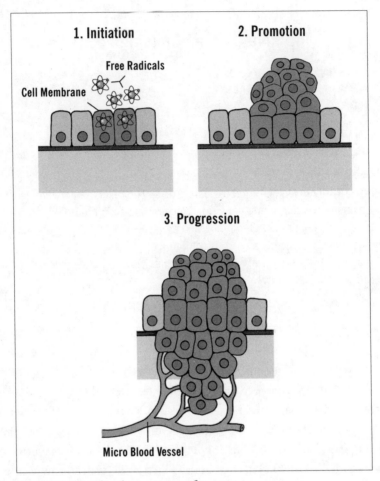

FIGURE 15 The three stages of cancer.

so called because there is no pain or indication of its presence growing in the body's organs.

It is at the initiation and promotion stages—before cancer has spread, or metastasized—that cancer is most curable. If Karen's cancer had been diagnosed when she first experienced abdominal pain and cramps, her outlook and response to treatment might have been much different.

Progression is cancer's final and most deadly stage. If all the body's defenses fail and a tumor begins to grow, it will start to release various growth factors to enhance its own survival. These growth factors stimulate surrounding healthy tissue to make thousands of new microscopic blood vessels to supply the cancerous growth—a process called *angiogenesis.* Without an ever-increasing blood supply, the tumor dies as its growth outpaces its nutrient supply. But with the development of new blood vessels, the tumor nourishes itself and acquires a pathway to seed other tumors elsewhere in the body.

After considering alternative cancer therapies and experimental clinical trials, Karen and her family selected an oncologist at a major cancer center, and she proceeded with conventional chemotherapy, which was not successful. At Karen's funeral, the tears and grief were overwhelming, as were my additional feelings of frustration and helplessness. I thought of the difficulty, and often futility, of trying to treat advanced cancer. As I knew only too well, the first and most significant line of defense against any cancer is to prevent it. With 1 in 4 people in the United States developing cancer, obviously we are not doing a great job at that. From hundreds of studies, we now know that various natural substances can neutralize free radicals, reduce the inflammatory response, and block angiogenesis, thus interfering with the three stages of cancer development. It's past time to turn that knowledge into action.

The use of compounds from plants in the treatment and prevention of many diseases predates recorded history. Modern medicine has continued to use plants themselves, such as foxglove, from which the heart drug digitalis is extracted, as well as to use biologically active plant molecules as a template for synthetic drugs. Between 2000 and 2005, more than twenty new anticancer drugs originating from plants or bacteria came on the market. One older example, Taxol, from the Pacific yew tree, is used for the treatment of breast, ovarian, and small-cell lung cancers.

Xeno Factors and Cancer

In 1979 Purdue University's Dr. John Pezzuto began a long, productive career investigating natural plant products that might inhibit or prevent cancer. After years of screening tens of thousands of compounds, in 1997 he and his team published a paper in the journal *Science* entitled "Cancer Chemopreventive Activity of Resveratrol, A Natural Product Derived from Grapes." For the first time, researchers demonstrated that a phytoalexin (a polyphenol xeno factor) could interfere with the three major stages of cancer production: it neutralized free radicals as an antioxidant in the initiation stage, acted as an anti-inflammatory during the promotion stage, and inhibited the formation of new blood vessels supplying the tumor during the progression stage. Pezzuto and his colleagues concluded their paper in the typically understated language of science researchers: "Our results suggest that resveratrol merits further investigation as a cancer chemopreventive agent in humans."

This publication sparked a huge response from other scientists, the media, and the public. Subsequently, hundreds of laboratories have investigated the molecular pathways and biological mechanisms of this and other polyphenols in relation to cancer protection (see list).

Cancers Inhibited by Resveratrol in Animals and Human Cell Models

Colon	Pancreas
Neuroblastoma	Ovary
Esophagus	Liver
Breast	Lung
Prostate	Stomach
Leukemia	Oral cavity
Metastasis to bone	Cervical
Squamous cell	Lymphoma
Melanoma	Thyroid

Thousands of scientific papers have been published, and companies have been formed to develop these new natural forms of cancer treatment and prevention. Xeno factors are now being evaluated for the treatment of many cancers: prostate, colon, lung, breast, ovary, kidney, liver, pancreas, skin, thyroid, and blood (leukemia). Although extremely complex, these studies support the initial indication that many natural xeno factors can act in potent ways to help prevent cancer. Even more relevant are studies in which xeno factors are tested in live animals and people.

Skin cancers, caused by overexposure to the sun, particularly ultraviolet B (UVB) radiation, are the most common cancer among humans. In a related animal study to determine whether resveratrol could decrease the damage caused by short-term UVB sun exposure, a single application of resveratrol was placed on the skin of hairless mice. This significantly blocked the increase in skin thickness and swelling typically seen with acute UVB sun exposure. There is now reason to believe that the xeno factor resveratrol may be the ultimate natural sunblock for both plants and animals, and may be useful in the treatment and prevention of some skin cancers.

Breast cancer, the most common cancer in women, represents 26 percent of all cancers and causes the death of forty thousand women in the United States each year. In one study, resveratrol was administered to mice by mouth starting seven days before they received a toxic agent that caused mammary cancer. After sixty-nine days of treatment, the incidence of cancer in the mice receiving resveratrol was reduced by approximately 50 percent. The investigators concluded that since resveratrol delayed the occurrence of mammary tumors and suppressed tumor formation at early stages, it might be more effective in the initiation and promotion stage than in the progressive stage.

Prostate cancer is the second most frequently diagnosed cancer, and its incidence increases significantly with men's age. Several xeno factors found in red grape skins, including catechin, epicatechin, quercetin, and resveratrol, have shown some effectiveness against prostate cancer. Grape skin extract, a rich source of resveratrol and other polyphenols, inhibited prostatic cancer growth up to 98 percent in a study on animals. It also has a direct action on the male hormone androgen, which is known to promote some forms of prostate cancer. In August 2007, scientists at the University of Alabama at Birmingham Comprehensive Cancer Center discovered a reduced incidence of prostate cancer in animals treated with resveratrol, as reported in the journal *Carcinogenesis.* They attributed this effect to the ability of resveratrol to interfere with tumor growth factors in the prostate.

Lung cancer accounts for approximately one-third of all cancer deaths in males and annually kills approximately 115,000 men and 100,000 women worldwide. Environmental factors such as smoking and pollution are the most important causes of lung cancer. As with breast cancer, studies using resveratrol and quercetin demonstrated that both had a significant effect on tumor growth and lung metastasis. In one group of animals, these xeno factors were administered for thirty-two days after implantation of malignant tumors. The results? Tumor growth was inhibited, and the formation of new capillaries at the site of the tumor was markedly reduced. When these xeno factors were administered into the abdominal cavity to treat tumor cells placed there, the compounds reduced tumor volume by 42 percent and metastasis to the lungs by 56 percent.

Colorectal cancer, which is responsible for approximately 10 percent of all U.S. cancer deaths in both men and women, kills approximately fifty thousand people per year. In another animal study, resveratrol was administered via oral fluids for one hundred days beginning ten days after administration of a colon cancer–inducing agent. Results suggested a definite protective effect by blocking DNA mutations, by activating immune cells, and by direct action on the genes that controlled cancer-cell proliferation and progression. Quercetin has also been studied, and it too showed specific oncogene-inhibiting effects.

Liver cancer, which is less common but still fatal in twenty thousand cases annually, was also investigated. As in the other studies, resveratrol reduced the incidence of solid tumor growth, decreased metastasis, and appeared to be preventive as well.

Further research on resveratrol has shown that it also has promise for treating pancreatic cancer. Dr. Paul Okunieff, chief of the department of radiation oncology at the University of Rochester Cancer Center, and his associates studied malignant human pancreatic cancer cells treated with and without resveratrol. They subjected the cells to ionizing radiation (radiation therapy). Their results were positive in two ways. First, resveratrol appeared to act as a tumor sensitizer: that is, it made the malignant cells more sensitive to radiation therapy. It also made normal tissue less sensitive to radiation, and this lower sensitivity would help minimize the treatment's adverse side effects. Second, the researchers believed that resveratrol enhanced the effects of chemotherapy. Both functions resulted in a higher kill rate of cancerous cells, a finding they reported in the March 2008 issue of the journal *Advances in Experimental Medicine and Biology.*

Looking at these and other studies, we can come to several conclusions:

- Xeno factors such as resveratrol, quercetin, and other compounds found in red grape skins demonstrate efficacy in preventing cancer in many animal models.
- These molecules block all three mechanisms of cancer formation—initiation, promotion, and progression—through their antioxidant, anti-inflammatory, and antiangiogenic effects.
- Effective treatment and prevention by xeno factors have been demonstrated in animals with cancers of the breast, skin, esophagus, colon, prostate, lung, and liver.

Human Cancer Studies

As we've seen, many of the cancer trials using xeno factors completed so far have dealt with either human cancer cell cultures (cells grown in a laboratory) or cancers found in certain animal models that resemble human cancers. These studies are required prior to any actual human trials of the effects of xeno factors on cancer. Currently, research led by Dr. David Boocock at England's University of Leicester is investigating oral doses of resveratrol (1.0, 2.5, or 5.0 g) in twenty-nine healthy human volunteers. This and other dosing studies will ultimately lead to human trials with cancer patients. Boocock and other researchers believe that the most promising cancer type to work with is human colon cancer, because the oral dose appears to be most concentrated in the gut. Other studies from other investigators will soon follow, using in-travenous dosing in a multitude of other cancer types.

In summary, a substantial body of laboratory and clinical research into the protective and therapeutic potential of resveratrol and other xeno factors suggests the following mechanisms for its benefits:

- Its anti-inflammatory effects, which inhibit the initial DNA mutations that lead to uncontrolled cell growth.
- Its promotion of the self-destruction of cancer cells through a process called *apoptosis*.
- Its inhibiting tumors from forming new blood vessels (antiangiogen-esis) to sustain themselves.
- Its inhibition of cancer cells, including those found in the lung, prostate, colon, liver, and skin, and in leukemias.

Now we can see why the discovery of xenohormesis may be one of the most significant breakthroughs in the prevention of cancer. Xeno-hormetic molecules from stressed plants—in particular stressed red grape skins—activate our sirtuin enzymes in the absence of caloric re-striction but with most of its benefits. Much needs to be learned about the molecular mechanisms by which sirtuin activation is cancer protec-tive, but the hundreds of studies done independently on the sirtuin genes and enzymes and now on xeno factors are converging.

Chapter 13

Stroke Prevention

Though nothing can bring back the hour of splendor in the grass, of glory in the flame; we will grieve not, rather find strength in what remains behind.

—WILLIAM WORDSWORTH

She was a coal miner's daughter, the "pick of the litter" of eleven kids, they said. Her father had been a salt miner in Poland; he immigrated just before the Great Depression to mine coal in eastern Ohio. He actually dug sixteen tons a day, and, as the song goes, did indeed owe his soul "to the company store." To save the soles of her shoes, she would walk barefoot to school and put the shoes on when she arrived. Her character, beauty, and goodness radiated for all to see.

Struggling in the hospital bed to speak words her brain couldn't find and being unable to walk due to paralysis in her right arm and leg were devastating to her—and to me. For many years before her stroke, I did my best to persuade my mother to stop smoking and not to join my father in his toxic diet. But she said, "Whither he goest, I too shall go." Unfortunately, she did. My mother's stroke, which eventually led to her demise, was like my father's heart attack—preventable. The triad of smoking, an inflammatory diet, and little or no physical exercise ended a beautiful life at age seventy-three.

The point of this and other stories in this book is that the diseases that rob us of our minds, our limbs, and our lives can be delayed or avoided entirely. Our bodies have been genetically modified by plants we've ingested over hundreds of thousands of years. As we've seen, when some of these natural plant products are ingested, they may act to prevent the development of cancer, heart disease, stroke, and Alzheimer's disease—the top four fatal diseases. In the case of my mother, we will look at how consuming xeno factors together with environmental and dietary changes might have lessened the effects of or even prevented her stroke.

Before describing the scientific studies on how xeno factors may help prevent strokes as well as reduce the devastating effects when strokes do occur, we need to have a rudimentary understanding of what is meant by a stroke. A stroke is the loss of function that results from cell death caused by a blockage or rupture in a blood vessel supplying oxygen to the brain. My mother was one of seven hundred thousand people a year in the United States who suffer a stroke. About five hundred thousand of these are first attacks. More women suffer strokes than men, perhaps because women live longer. Approximately 1 in 8 stroke victims will die with the first attack.

The word *stroke* comes from the ancient Greeks, who believed that the suddenness of the affliction was a sign that the victim had been "struck" down by the gods. Although most occur abruptly, some may be preceded by episodes called transient ischemic attacks (TIAs), in which there is temporary loss of blood flow for minutes or hours.

Because a stroke is similar to a heart attack—both are forms of vascular, or blood circulation, disease—it is now commonly referred to as a "brain attack." This means that the same five stages of development of a blood clot apply to ischemic strokes, the type that involve blockage: (1) the accumulation of fat and free radicals, (2) the subsequent inflammatory response and impaired tone of the blood vessel, (3) the increase in platelets at the site of injury, (4) the resultant clotting, and (5) the damage to the brain.

The word *ischemic* is derived from the Greek word for "keeping back," or blocking, blood flow to a specific area. An ischemic stroke usually develops in the carotid arteries in the neck, which supply blood to the brain. These strokes can occur because the walls of the artery thicken until the flow abruptly stops. Or they strike when plaque in the carotid arteries breaks off and is forced into the smaller blood vessels of the brain, blocking the blood supply to a specific portion of the brain.

If the blockage occurs in a large blood vessel supplying the brain, as it did with my mother, a large part of the brain may be suddenly damaged, with devastating consequences. Many elderly people, however, experience a series of what are called ministrokes. This is caused by blockage of small blood vessels, often aggravated by high blood pressure. The consequences, over time, may be memory impairment or even dementia.

The second major type of brain attack is called a hemorrhagic stroke. It is caused not by a blood clot but by a blood vessel rupturing. This occurs much less frequently than the blockage type of stroke, but it also usually stems from degeneration of blood vessels due to *arteriosclerosis,* or hardening.

The top risk factors for blockage strokes include arteriosclerosis, high blood pressure, excessive blood-clotting factors, diabetes (which can result in chronic inflammation of the blood vessel walls), heart valve defects, and aging. Many factors predispose us to brain attacks. The nicotine and carbon monoxide in cigarette smoke directly damage the lining of blood vessels and cause blood vessels to constrict. Heredity also plays a major role; the chance of a stroke is much greater in those who have a family history of strokes. African Americans also have a much higher risk of stroke and of disability from stroke than Caucasians. This is partly because they have a greater incidence of hypertension. Elevated blood pressure is the most prominent risk factor for a stroke, so reducing blood pressure is a primary preventive measure.

Unlike the heart, in which muscle is damaged, the brain has two major zones of injury associated with a stroke. The first is the core zone, the part where virtually no blood supply gets to the cells. Neurons (nerve cells) in this zone die within a few minutes of oxygen deprivation, resulting in immediate loss of function (see figure 16).

A second major zone of injury borders the area of tissue death like a halo. This region, underoxygenated and electrically silent, but still alive, is called the ischemic penumbra. (*Penumbra* comes from the

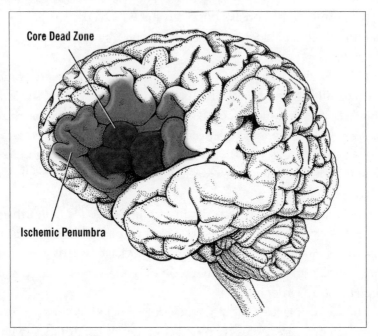

Core Dead Zone

Ischemic Penumbra

FIGURE 16 Post-stroke brain showing the dead area and the ischemic penumbra with its nonfunctioning cells, which are potentially revivable.

Latin word for "shadow.") A major goal of acute stroke management is to quickly resuscitate the patient and reestablish blood flow and oxygen to the penumbra brain tissue. This is where pharmacological interventions, such as clot-busting drugs and surgery to remove clots and repair blood vessels, do their work. Unfortunately, the window of opportunity for brain resuscitation after a brain attack is relatively short.

My mother, who lived alone, had her stroke soon after waking up in the morning and did not get to the hospital for more than three hours. She had an immediate CT scan of her brain, which showed no hemorrhage (that is, no blood outside the vessels). She then had an angiogram to visualize the arteries in her neck and brain, which revealed an acute blockage due to a blood clot in the left carotid artery in her neck. For her it was too late.

What to Do If You Suspect Someone Has Suffered a Stroke

Call 911 immediately. Remember to act FAST:

F=Face. Ask the person to smile. Does one side of the face droop?

A=Arms. Ask the person to raise both arms. Does one arm drift downward?

S=Speech. Ask the person to repeat a simple sentence. Are the words slurred? Can the person repeat the sentence correctly?

T=Time. If the person shows any of these symptoms, time is important. Call 911 or get to the hospital fast. Brain cells are dying.

SOURCE: NATIONAL STROKE ASSOCIATION.

Xeno Factors and Brain Protection

As we have emphasized throughout this book, the old adage rings true: An ounce of prevention is worth a pound of cure. Xeno factors are known to significantly help prevent atherosclerosis and clot formation within blood vessels in animals. Their effects as an antioxidant, an anti-inflammatory, a blood vessel dilator, and an inhibitor of clot formation all should contribute to a reduction in brain attacks.

Knowing that xeno factors help the heart recover from the injury of a heart attack, scientists were curious about the ability of these compounds to protect the brain before and after a brain attack. Numerous studies both with cultured brain cells and in live animals have now demonstrated that various xeno factors can protect animals' brain cells. In animals pretreated with resveratrol, paralysis from a stroke was prevented, and the size of the brain injury was decreased. In another study, pretreatment and concurrent treatment with resveratrol significantly reduced the size of dead tissue in rats after major brain artery blockage.

In January 2007, neurosurgical investigators at Inönü University in Turkey extrapolated from the above studies a concept of neuronal protection and further investigated the effect of resveratrol in traumatic brain injury. They divided albino male rats with brain trauma into three groups—an untreated control group and two treatment groups—using different doses of resveratrol. They concluded that resveratrol administered immediately after a traumatic brain injury decreased the amount of free-radical damage and also significantly reduced the area of tissue damage.

Investigators have also found that resveratrol may be neuroprotective in the spinal cord following injury. In 2004 researcher Ugursay Kiziltepe reported in the *Journal of Vascular Surgery* that resveratrol protected the spinal cord from damage by enhancing energy metabolism and decreasing the injury to axons and myelin. Axons, the projections from a nerve cell, connect with other neurons and are insulated by a white material called myelin.

Nationally, 1.4 million people sustain traumatic brain injury each year, mostly from car accidents and other mishaps. Of these, 50,000 will die and 235,000 are hospitalized. Another 10,000 suffer severe spinal cord damage.

The potential mechanisms of neuroprotection from xeno factors are very similar to those in the heart. The antioxidant activity and the scavenging of free radicals, the effect of decreasing inflammation, and more recently, the discovery of the activation of the SIRT1 enzyme all have been suggested to contribute to these neuroprotective and brain-sparing effects.

The best approach, however, is still prevention. Strong scientific data confirm that xenohormetic molecules from stressed plants activate specific genes that provide neuroprotection to the brain and play a major role in preventing and ameliorating the effects of a brain attack. Taking xeno factors regularly is now being intensely investigated for its preventive and protective effects, as we will now see in other neurological diseases.

Chapter 14

Degenerative Brain Diseases and Brain Protection

Resveratrol is not only neuroprotective, it also improves cognitive function after neurodegeneration.

—LI-HUEI TSAI, PROFESSOR OF NEUROSCIENCE
AT MIT, 2007

Auguste Deter was the happily married wife of an office clerk until midway into her fifty-second year. One day she observed her husband taking a walk with a neighbor friend and became atypically jealous. From then on, her relationship with her husband became very cool, as did her relationship with the neighbor. Soon after, she began to have difficulty remembering where she put things. Her house, which she had maintained meticulously, became disheveled. While preparing meals, which had always been a pleasant chore, she became confused about the ingredients. She paced nervously for no reason and was no longer careful with the household money.

The changes in Auguste Deter progressively worsened. She slowly became paranoid, sure that other people's conversations were about her. A familiar local deliveryman suddenly seemed dangerous. She developed a terrible fear of dying and would become so agitated that she would tremble. The confusion and disorientation progressed to the point where she would ring her neighbors' doorbells for no apparent reason.

Over the next four years, Auguste Deter's memory deteriorated until it was totally erased. She became apathetic and was confined to bed, her legs drawn up in the fetal position. Unable to control her bowels or bladder, she suffered from major ulcers and skin breakdown on her lower back and hips. Infection ensued, pneumonia developed, and she died on April 7, 1906, in the Hospital for the Mentally Ill and Epileptic in Frankfurt, Germany.

When Mrs. Deter was first committed to the hospital on November 25, 1901, she was assigned to a young doctor who had begun his residency in psychiatry three years before. His name was Alois Alzheimer. After studying medicine in Berlin, Würzburg, and Tübingen, Alzheimer graduated from medical school with highest honors in 1888. To earn extra money and travel, he accepted a job accompanying a mentally ill woman on a journey that lasted five months. Observing her, he became obsessed with the mechanisms of mental illness and the bizarre behavior that developed in previously normal people.

Once his travels ended, he joined the faculty of the insane asylum to which Mrs. Deter would be admitted, to work under Emil Sioli, an open-minded, liberal psychiatrist. Although Alzheimer was studying psychiatry, he was also very fond of working with the microscope to study the cortex of the human brain. There was no lack of patients to observe. At the turn of the century, the number of mentally ill patients was rapidly increasing in Germany. Sexually transmitted diseases that affect the brain, like syphilis, were widespread, and the number of patients with neuropsychiatric complications was on the rise.

Before the late 1800s, dementia was thought to be caused by divine retribution. Alzheimer and other scientists in Germany were in the vanguard of those who would confirm that mental illness was not God's punishment for moral transgressions. Rather, they discovered that loss of memory, cognition, and judgment, as well as depression, pathological anxiety, and fear, all had underlying anatomical and biochemical causes found in the brain.

It was in this environment that Alzheimer first met Auguste Deter. After working with her for two years and meticulously documenting her deterioration, he moved to Munich, where he became renowned for his description of the neuropathology of patients with mental illness and progressive paralysis.

When Alzheimer learned of Mrs. Deter's death, he immediately requested that his former professor, Dr. Sioli, open her skull, remove her brain, and ship it to Munich for study. When he first lifted it out of the formaldehyde, he immediately saw that it was approximately half the weight of a normal brain. The outer cortex (from the Latin for "bark") was shrunken, so that the normal grooves, or sulci, were much more prominent than normal.

The next step, one that he had performed thousands of times with other brains, was the most important. Using a very long knife, similar to one used on wedding cakes, he cut the brain crosswise into approximately twenty slices. He then took small sections from the shrunken temporal lobes, responsible for memory, and from the frontal lobes, which serve the executive functions of cognition, analysis, and mental states. He stained them with special dyes, observed them under a microscope, and recorded his observations.

Where neurons had once been located, he saw tangled nerve fibers, which he dubbed "neurofibrillary tangles." He also saw an accumulation of clumps of a starchlike substance called *amyloid,* again signaling destruction of neurons. These observations of tangles and plaques confirmed for the very first time the correlation between changes in the brain and the mental disease that he had so meticulously and personally documented in Mrs. Deter.

After her death, Alzheimer gave a report on the case at a conference of psychiatrists in Tübingen. The title of his lecture was "On a Peculiar Disease of the Cerebral Cortex." Subsequently, his chairman of psychiatry in Munich, Emil Kraepelin, suggested that this "presenile dementia," with its diffuse shrinkage of the brain, changes in the inner structure, and death of neurons, be called Alzheimer's disease (AD).

As with many great discoveries in medicine, it would take decades before the true significance of Alzheimer's observation took hold. In fact, it wasn't until the 1970s that his work was "rediscovered." With the aging of the American population, dementia was becoming an epidemic. Around that time, Parkinson's disease was linked to a deficiency in dopamine, a neurotransmitter in the brain. This led to the discovery that Alzheimer's disease was related to a deficiency in the neurotransmitter acetylcholine (ACH). Healthy ACH levels are critically important for memory formation and retention. Various discoveries about the way neurotransmitters modulate behavior have led to a new conceptualization of mental illness, laying the groundwork for modern biological psychiatry. The present drugs approved for treating Alzheimer's increase acetylcholine or its effectiveness.

Over the last twenty years, Alzheimer's disease has come to be regarded as a genetic disease. With the use of modern tools of molecular biology such as electron microscopy (which uses electrons rather than visible light to highly magnify tissue), the connection between gene activation through what we ingest (nutrigenomics) and many diseases like Alzheimer's is now becoming clearer. So our next question becomes this: might a known gene activating product containing natural xeno factors play a role in moderating a genetically related disease like Alzheimer's? Once again, the primary emphasis is on prevention, for as an ancient Chinese metaphor puts it, "To fight a disease after it has occurred is like trying to dig a well when one is thirsty or forging a weapon once a war has begun." In the case of Alzheimer's disease, complete prevention would be ideal, but even success in delaying onset or reducing the severity of this devastating disease would benefit millions.

We know that the prevalence of Alzheimer's disease increases with age. For those under sixty-five, there is less than a 5 percent chance of developing Alzheimer's unless one has the specific genes that account for approximately 2 percent to 5 percent of the cases. After age sixty-five, however, there is a 1 in 108 chance of developing this form of brain degeneration. And after age eighty-five, it is estimated that half the population will die from Alzheimer's if they live long enough. Alzheimer's is by far the most common cause of dementia among those over age sixty-five, currently afflicting approximately 4.5 million people in the United States. It is the fourth-leading cause of death after heart disease, cancer, and stroke. The message of Alzheimer's is clear: it is not enough to live longer; we must also live healthier.

As if the human toll were not great enough, the economic expense of Alzheimer's is also horrendous. Close to one million people with the disease now reside in nursing homes, where, with good medical care, patients can live eight to twelve years before dying with brains incapable of remembering the past. The annual treatment costs in the United States are approximately $100 billion, but, of course, the devastating effects on the individual and the family are incalculable.

Triggers of Alzheimer's Disease

Over the past fifteen years or so, evidence has accumulated that Alzheimer's disease is also a chronic, inflammatory process in the brain. Evidence for this inflammatory component is twofold. First, around

Diagnosis of Alzheimer's Disease

Alzheimer's disease is, generally speaking, initially identified in only half of affected patients. The symptoms are subtle and are often associated with an umbrella diagnosis of "old age." Since there is as yet no definitive diagnostic test for Alzheimer's, it is critically important to rule out other brain diseases. Imaging the brain with a CT scan or, preferably, a magnetic resonance imaging (MRI) scan, is an important screening tool for other conditions. More recently, the FDG-PET scan (fluorodeoxyglucose-positron emission tomography) has shown promise in detecting the abnormal changes in the brain that take place with Alzheimer's. Scientists at the University of Pittsburgh recently discovered a compound called the Pittsburgh Compound-B (PIB), which, when injected into a vein, can enhance amyloid deposits in the brain tissue on PET scans of living patients. A clinical trial reported in the *New England Journal of Medicine* in 2007 confirmed this as the first definitive neuroimaging test to diagnose Alzheimer's disease in a living patient.

the amyloid plaques described by Alois Alzheimer, researchers have found a sharp increase in white blood cells and inflammatory cytokines responsible for inflammation. Second, there are approximately twenty population studies indicating that nonsteroidal anti-inflammatory drugs like Celebrex, ibuprofen, and others reduce the age-related prevalence of Alzheimer's disease. There are also several studies in which patients who were placed on aspirin, as recommended by their doctors for heart disease, had a lower incidence of Alzheimer's as they got older.

So why aren't these anti-inflammatories the silver bullets for treating Alzheimer's? Unfortunately, at this time we do not know why some people are protected and others are not. We do know from genetic testing that some people are clearly more predisposed to developing the disease than others. If a patient tests positive for genetic factors but is asymptomatic, this is an ideal scenario for the use of anti-

Alzheimer's Disease Risk Factors

Major risk factors for developing Alzheimer's disease (AD), as mentioned, are advancing age and a family history of the disease. You are 25 percent more likely than the rest of the population to develop early AD if one of your parents has the early-onset form of the disease. Having more years of formal education has been found in some studies to reduce AD risk. This effect may be due to increased brain cell function or the fact that the density of these brain cell connections (synapses) may be increased if the mind is kept active as we age. Other factors, such as unemployment, obesity, and inflammatory dietary factors like trans-fatty acids, have all been linked to various degrees of greater risk. Specifically, high intake of dietary fat may increase the risk of AD, whereas fish and whole grains have shown to reduce the risk. Generally, diets that promote inflammation have been shown to contribute to the development of AD. Diets that can reduce inflammation, or taking specific supplements to reduce free radical production and inflammation, can provide a reduction in risk for the development of AD. These supplements include vitamin C, vitamin E, beta-carotene, and especially fish oil.

inflammatories, xeno factors, and the reduction of other risk factors to help prevent or delay Alzheimer's disease.

Cardiovascular disease appears to be a major risk factor for the subsequent development of Alzheimer's disease. Recent scientific evidence indicates that the likelihood of Alzheimer's disease (as well as stroke) is greatly increased in patients with heart disease. In fact, these three diseases—heart disease, stroke, and Alzheimer's—are referred to as "the deadly triad." Studies show that elderly survivors of heart disease and stroke subsequently develop Alzheimer's disease at a much greater rate than normal. When the brain does not receive enough oxygen—a condition called hypoxia, which is common in patients with heart disease—this may trigger the development of Alzheimer's disease. A recent report from the New York Academy of Sciences indicated that hypoxia activates a gene called BACE1. This specific gene is known to produce the *amyloid-beta* plaques that Dr. Alzheimer initially found in the brains of Alzheimer's patients (see figure 17).

Xeno Factors and Brain Protection

In September 2006 Thimmappa S. Anekonda from the Neurological Science Institute at the Oregon Health and Science University published an article in *Brain Research Reviews* entitled "Resveratrol— A Boon for Treating Alzheimer's Disease?" Drawing on the work of Guarente, Sinclair, Baur, and many others, he summarized why sirtuin-activating compounds like resveratrol are potent agents for neuroprotection against Alzheimer's disease and stroke in the brain, focusing on their ability to reduce damage to the mitochondria—the cell's power plants.

In the development of Alzheimer's disease, it is thought that the accumulation of free radicals may activate an enzyme, beta-secretase, which results in formation of the amyloid-beta protein. This protein itself is toxic and inflammatory. In the brain, supporting cells to neurons called microglia act as scavengers in much the same fashion as white blood cells do in the bloodstream. They engulf and attempt to eliminate the dead neurons initially damaged by the free radicals. Unfortu-

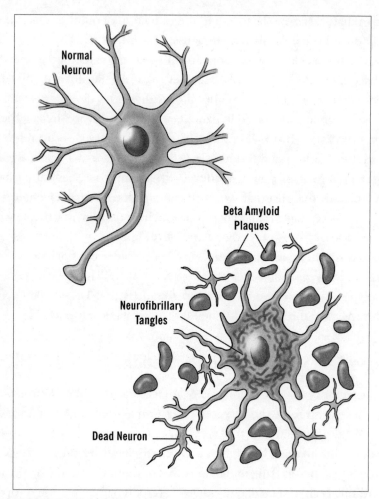

FIGURE 17 Alzheimer's plaques and tangles.

nately, they also manufacture harmful toxic agents as well as additional free radicals in their attempt to eliminate the dead cells. These toxins break down cellular membranes and damage mitochondria, and the cascade effect results in dementia and death.

Many scientists have now shown that resveratrol influences and may block the production of the free radicals that set in motion these destructive processes. In one study, human umbilical vein cells were challenged with the amyloid-beta toxic substance. When nutrients containing resveratrol and quercetin as well as vitamins E and C were introduced, they protected these cells from free radical damage, reduced the production of free radicals, and prevented cellular DNA damage. In other studies, resveratrol protected neurons in the hippocampus (the memory center) from nitric oxide toxicity, another destructive molecule in the inflammatory process. Several other studies confirmed these results both in cell cultures and in animals. Interestingly, resveratrol exhibited its positive effects whether it was used as a pretreatment, a cotreatment, or a posttreatment.

Another way that resveratrol provides protection from Alzheimer's disease is by facilitating the removal of the toxic amyloid-beta substances, or plaques. Proteosomes are proteins that serve as quality-control mechanisms in the brain. They degrade and remove deformed proteins. Because of the plethora of abnormal proteins in Alzheimer's disease, the proteosome system becomes overwhelmed. In experimental studies, resveratrol directly reduced the levels of the amyloid-beta plaques, using mechanisms similar to that of proteosomes.

There are several other neurodegenerative diseases in which SIRT1 may have therapeutic potential. In March 2008 Lenny Guarente, at the Pasteur Institute in Paris, presented his new data on Huntington's disease, a devastating neurodegenerative condition associated with premature mental and physical deterioration. He showed that mice lived longer and had less disease in the brain when SIRT1 was increased. Other investigators have found neuroprotective effects in animals bred to have amyotrophic lateral sclerosis (Lou Gehrig's disease), and also in optic neuritis, which leads to blindness. According to Christoph Westphal, MD, the CEO of Sirtris Pharmaceuticals, "These neuroprotective data expand the promise for small molecule sirtuin activators as potential therapeutics for a broad range of disease of aging."

All of these neuroprotective studies in both Alzheimer's and stroke circle back to observations of the ways that calorie restriction and sirtuin activating compounds—the xeno factor—promote longevity and healthy aging. By activating genes and enzymes, in particular SIRT1, xeno factors do indeed confer neuronal protection. Under-

Other Natural Anti-inflammatories

It is no surprise that consumption of fish oil (omega-3 fatty acids), one of the best natural anti-inflammatories, has been shown to slow the development of Alzheimer's disease. Major epidemiological studies have confirmed that the higher the fish or fish oil consumption in different population groups, the lower the chance of developing Alzheimer's. In 2007 the National Institutes of Health took the next step, launching a fifty-one-site study to determine if fish oil given to patients with early signs of Alzheimer's disease can reduce the risk of cognitive decline. The results won't be conclusive for five to ten years, but scientists are hopeful.

standing of this mechanism is still in its infancy, but resveratrol-induced SIRT1 activation has been shown to protect neurons in animal models of Huntington's disease—a terrible congenital condition characterized by brain degeneration, dementia, and abnormal movements. In studies of Parkinson's disease, protection was conferred by delaying degeneration of axons, the parts of the neuron responsible for transmiting impulses from one neuron to the next. These and other studies strongly implicate sirtuins in nerve protection and show that xeno factors can elevate sirtuin production in the human brain.

Chapter 15

Other Inflammatory Conditions

Because of xeno factors' potent anti-inflammatory effects, scientists around the world are beginning to study their potential benefit in a host of diseases associated with rampant inflammation. These include severe lung disease, colitis, arthritis, and alcohol-induced hepatitis. Let's look at some of these individually.

Chronic Obstructive Pulmonary Disease (COPD)

Chronic obstructive pulmonary disease (COPD) is an umbrella term for chronic bronchitis, emphysema, and a range of other lung disorders. Around 90 percent of cases are due to smoking tobacco, but I have seen it in my own patients from coal dust, asbestos, and industrial solvents. I witnessed the progressive and devastating symptoms in my mother—a chronic smoker—over the course of approximately twenty years. It begins with shortness of breath often associated with wheezing, and eventually a persistent cough. As it progresses to the severe stage, a bluish discoloration is seen in the lips and fingers: this is due to the lack of oxygen in the blood.

Emphysema is the most common type of COPD. Smoke of any kind damages the elasticity of the lung tissue that supports the alveoli, or air sacs, through which oxygen and carbon dioxide diffuse. These millions of tiny sacs surrounded by capillaries in the lungs absorb oxygen and transfer it into the blood. Toxins such as smoke get trapped in the alveoli and result in a profound inflammatory response. This inflammation is every bit as destructive as an open wound.

According to the World Health Organization, eighty million people suffer from moderate to severe COPD, and three million died of it in 2005. It is considered the fourth-greatest cause of death worldwide. Treatment is multifaceted. It includes giving up smoking and, if necessary, changing jobs. Drug therapy encompasses a laundry list of medications called bronchodilators, which relax the smooth muscles of the airway, improving blood flow. Of prime importance are drugs that reduce inflammation in the lungs, such as corticosteroids, taken in pill form or combined with inhalers.

Enter Xeno Factors

Researchers at Imperial College in London, England, studied the anti-inflammatory action of red wine ingredients on white blood cells involved in the inflammatory process in patients with COPD. They compared lung fluid samples taken from smokers and nonsmokers and found that resveratrol more than halved the production of the harmful inflammatory factors that result in the coughing, wheezing, and destruction of lung tissue. Lead researcher Louise Donnelly said, "Resveratrol exhibited anti-inflammatory activity in all the systems we examined, including laboratory cell lines as well as real human airway epithelial cells."

Dr. Donnelly also concluded that resveratrol and quercetin found in red wine might be beneficial when steroids have proved ineffective in inflammatory diseases, such as COPD, steroid-resistant asthma, and arthritis. She ended by saying, "These compounds may provide candidate molecules for the development of novel anti-inflammatory therapies." Inhalants and aerosols are under investigation. Dr. John Harvey of the British Thoracic Society supported the potential benefit of resveratrol by saying, "It seems like drinking red wine in moderation as part of a healthy, balanced diet can reduce lung inflammation," and hence COPD.

Even more exciting is the potential benefit of the sirtuin gene and resveratrol in smokers with COPD and/or lung cancer. Dr. Irfan Rahman, associate professor of environmental medicine at the University of Rochester Medical Center Lung Biology and Disease Program, has studied how the 4,700 toxic chemical compounds in cigarettes assault lung tissue. In collaboration with Vuokko L. Kinnula, MD, at the University of Helsinki in Finland, he studied the levels of SIRT1 in the lungs of nonsmokers and smokers with and without COPD. Thirty-seven patients from Helsinki who were undergoing either lung removal surgery for suspected cancer or a lung transplant volunteered to provide tissue samples. These researchers confirmed that SIRT1 was significantly reduced in smokers compared with nonsmokers. They discovered that the sirtuin gene plays a major role in regulating the chemical signaling system that protects the lungs from smoke and pollution.

These investigators have already taken the next step in exploring the potential of the powerful antioxidant and anti-inflammatory abilities of resveratrol to reverse lung damage in patients with COPD. Dr. Rahman concluded, "The hallmark of this discovery [the sirtuin gene–resveratrol connection] is that we may be able to provide remedies to millions of smokers who would like to quit but cannot kick their addiction, and millions of former smokers who, despite quitting, remain at risk for illness as they age."

Colitis

Colitis literally means inflammation of the colon, or large intestine. The term is used to refer to any number of colon disorders presenting symptoms of diarrhea (often with blood and mucus), abdominal pain, and fever. Ulcerative colitis is another inflammatory disease of the colon associated with ulceration of the lining of the colon and rectum. Crohn's disease is a form of colitis that involves thickening of the intestinal wall. It typically occurs in the small intestine, near the point where it joins the large colon, but the colon and other parts of the gastrointestinal track may be affected as well. The term *inflammatory bowel disease (IBD)* refers to both ulcerative colitis and Crohn's disease, as well as to a less severe disorder called irritable bowel syndrome (IBS).

Chances are good that you know someone with IBD. It affects as many as two million people in the United States. For unknown reasons, it is especially common in people of Jewish descent and is rarely seen in Eastern Europe, Asia, and South America. It is also rare in the African-American population. Although the causes of IBD are unknown, we know that it involves an intense inflammatory reaction mediated by white blood cells. It is characterized by a marked increase in free radicals and various inflammatory signaling factors, much like COPD.

In 2006 Dr. Antonio Ramón Martín and his associates at Spain's University of Seville published, in the *British Journal of Pharmacology,* a study in which they injected an irritant that produced intense IBD-like symptoms in laboratory animals. They gave the treatment group resveratrol for two weeks, and then compared the degree of inflammation in the treated and untreated groups. The untreated animals suffered from weight loss, diarrhea, and evidence of marked inflammation and ulcerations of the large intestine. In the group given resveratrol, as compared with the untreated group, damage was reduced markedly: the ulcers were in the process of healing, and the number of factors causing inflammation was dramatically reduced. Dr. Martín and his associates concluded, "We have shown that resveratrol exerts protective effects in chronic experimental colitis. These and our previous results strongly suggest the use of resveratrol in controlling IBD."

Disease affecting the intestines and liver may provide the very best targets for orally ingested xeno factors, since one concern with oral ingestion is the legitimate question of how much of the active compound gets into the bloodstream. These polyphenols have direct action and contact with the intestine and then are transported to the liver, so for the intestine and liver, the respective concentrations would be very high and therefore probably more beneficial. Again, human trials are needed to evaluate true efficacy.

Liver Protection from Excess Alcohol

The liver weighs about three pounds and is located in the upper right-hand side of the abdominal cavity, just beneath the rib cage. It regulates chemical levels in the blood and excretes bile, which helps to break down fats for further digestion and absorption. All the products of digestion that leave the stomach and intestine pass through the liver. Here the nutrients and drugs that we ingest are broken down into forms that can be used by the rest of the body.

The liver performs more than five hundred vital functions, including:

- Producing cholesterol and special proteins to carry fats throughout the body
- Converting excess sugar into glycogen for storage
- Regulating blood levels of amino acids, which form the building blocks of proteins
- Clearing the blood of drugs and other poisonous substances
- Regulating blood clotting
- Producing immune factors and removing bacteria from the bloodstream

Studies show that one or two average-sized alcoholic drinks per day may help prevent heart disease and stroke, as well as other conditions. When this level is exceeded, however, there is a likelihood of developing three types of liver conditions: fatty liver, hepatitis, and cirrhosis. Hepatitis, or inflammation of the liver, ranges from mild to severe, and can impair or destroy many essential liver functions. In general, the amount and duration of alcohol excess correlate with the presence and severity of liver damage. Still, only 20 percent to 30 percent of long-term alcohol abusers suffer severe liver disease. One study estimated that cirrhosis develops in only 14 percent of alcoholics consuming twelve drinks per day for eight years.

Because of the high incidence of alcoholism in Spain, investigators were intrigued by the weak correlation between the larger amount of alcohol consumed by Spaniards and the notable reduction of liver disease in that country. They explored the possibility that one or more environmental factors might be mitigating the effect of alcohol on the livers of heavy-drinking Spaniards. Specifically, they wondered whether the resveratrol in wine, through its anti-inflammatory effects in the body, might actually protect against liver damage.

To answer this question, they devised an experiment. They divided laboratory animals into four groups: (1) rats not given alcohol, (2) rats not given alcohol but treated with resveratrol, (3) rats given alcohol, and (4) rats given alcohol and treated with resveratrol. The animals subjected to alcohol intoxication without resveratrol showed poor general health after the second week, reflected by decreased activity levels, immobility, and coarse hair. No such differences were observed in the other three groups. Investigators speculated that the reduced mortality in the fourth group was related to the antioxidant, anti-inflammatory, and anti-infectious properties of resveratrol.

Luis Bujand, the lead author, from the department of genetics at the Basurto Hospital in Bilbao, Spain, concluded: "Resveratrol reduces mortality and liver damage produced by alcohol in mice. If our findings are confirmed by further research, resveratrol could be administered to patients with chronic alcoholism to reduce the mortality and liver damage associated with alcohol abuse." He and his associates went on to say, "It could even be prophylactically added to alcoholic beverages, similar to the way chlorine is added to water to prevent infections."

Arthritis

Arthritis (from the Greek word *arthro,* or joint, and *-itis,* or inflammation) refers to a group of conditions that damage the joints of the body. Arthritis is the leading cause of disability in people over the age of fifty-five. There are many forms, each with a different cause. The two most common types are osteoarthritis and rheumatoid arthritis.

Osteoarthritis, often called degenerative arthritis, is a condition in which low-grade inflammation due to normal wear and tear brings about pain in the joints. Usually the cartilage that covers the joints wears down, causing pain during weight-bearing activities such as walking and standing. This condition affects approximately twenty-one million people in the United States and accounts for 25 percent of visits to primary care physicians. Treatment includes nonsteroidal anti-inflammatories, local injections of corticosteroids, and in severe cases, joint replacement.

Rheumatoid arthritis, on the other hand, is a chronic inflammatory disease in which the body literally attacks itself, making this an autoimmune disorder. It often involves swelling in many joints at the same time (polyarthritis). The pain is usually worst in the morning, in contrast to the pain of osteoarthritis, which gets worse over the course of the day. Rheumatoid arthritis is also associated with anemia and deformities of the joints, particularly the hands and feet. In both types of arthritis, inflammation is the major cause of pain, swelling, and joint destruction.

Because of its potent anti-inflammatory effect, resveratrol is being investigated by scientists around the world for its potential in treating arthritis. In October 2007, investigators at Germany's University of Munich reported their work on the regulation of inflammation in cartilage cells taken from the knees of human patients. They found that resveratrol exhibited a potent anti-inflammatory effect.

Scientists in Turkey evaluated the effects of resveratrol on chemically induced inflammatory arthritis in animals. They injected irritant material directly into the joints of anesthetized animals and confirmed cartilage destruction in the control group. Those animals treated with resveratrol injected directly into the inflamed joints showed only mild to moderate inflammation compared with the damaged control group. The authors of the study postulated that the reduced inflammation resulted in the improvement. They concluded, "Resveratrol may provide a novel and alternative approach as a disease-modifying agent in the progression of inflammatory arthritis."

Although further clinical trials are needed, resveratrol, together with other natural anti-inflammatory compounds, may be able, in certain situations, to replace powerful pharmaceutical drugs, which have attendant side effects.

More than half of the patients I see in my neurosurgical practice suffer from pain due to degenerative arthritis and complications such as ruptured or herniated disks and spinal stenosis (narrowing of the spinal canal). Virtually all are taking nonsteroidal anti-inflammatories like Advil (ibuprofen), the COX-2 inhibitor Celebrex (celecoxib), Aleve (naproxen), aspirin, and many more. Unfortunately, these are associated with complications such as bleeding ulcers, heart attacks, and strokes. After experiencing a gastric ulcer myself from overuse of ibuprofen I was taking for arthritis in my knee, I investigated natural anti-inflammatories that could possibly serve as a substitute. I discovered that fish oil, with its omega-3 fatty acids, was one of the very best natural anti-inflammatories and also reduced pain. After taking regular doses of fish oil, I was able to stop taking anti-inflammatories altogether.

Impressed with the powerful effect of this natural substance, I decided to conduct a study in my own patients to assess its effectiveness. I took 250 patients who were on Vioxx, Celebrex, Bextra, or Ibuprofen and put them on high doses of pharmaceutical-grade fish oil. Two-thirds were able to give up the pharmaceutical drugs and instead take fish oil as their anti-inflammatory. We published our results in *Surgical Neurology,* a peer-reviewed journal, in 2007.

I looked into the mechanism through which fish oil was effective and discovered that it worked along the same pathways as resveratrol. Both block the nuclear factor kappa B transcription factors that lead to inflammation. They thus reduce pain, swelling, and inflammation. Now I recommend that my patients take a combination of pharmaceutical-grade fish oil (see appendix D) and resveratrol almost to the exclusion of nonsteroidal anti-inflammatories.

Chapter 16

Sources, Safety, Bioavailability, and Dosage

The three stages of truth for scientists: (1) It's not true. (2) If it is true, it's not very important. (3) We knew it all along.
—LEO SZILARD, PHYSICIST ON THE MANHATTAN PROJECT

In the last few pages, we walked through some of the extensive data linking resveratrol and other polyphenols to prevention and possible treatment of a host of chronic diseases. Now let's take a look at the sources of these bioactive molecules; their stability, absorption (bioavailability), and safety; and suggested dosages for effectiveness.

Natural Sources

Resveratrol

As we've discussed, plants produce specialized protective polyphenol compounds called phytoalexins when they are stressed by parasites, various infections, ultraviolet radiation, or injury. Resveratrol, a potent phytoalexin, was originally identified in 1940 from the white hellebore lily. The most concentrated natural source of resveratrol is the Asian medicinal plant *Polygonum cuspidatum* (giant knotweed), which the Japanese call *ko-jo-kon* and the Chinese call *fo-ti* or *ho shou wu*. Resveratrol, together with other bioactive ingredients in these plants, has been used for thousands of years in traditional Chinese and Indian medicines.

In the human diet, the greatest source of resveratrol and associated polyphenols is the skins of red grapes, which use resveratrol to ward off attacks, particularly from fungi. During winemaking, this resveratrol becomes concentrated. The type of grape, climate, and soil are all factors that influence the level of resveratrol found in a given red wine. The most important element is how long the skins are kept in contact with the fermenting juice during the winemaking process. The longer the contact, the higher the resveratrol content. Even though some white wines are made from grapes with a high phytoalexin content, the skin is removed sooner for color purposes, giving these wines a much lower resveratrol concentration than red wines. Rosé wines (a combination of red and white grapes), as would be expected, have a midlevel concentration (see table 6 on page 150).

Some winegrowers are now beginning to produce resveratrol as a commercial product, inducing plants to produce greater quantities by adding stressors to the grape shoots and vines. Also, red grapes exposed to ultraviolet UVB sunlight and ultraviolet UVC radiation, which is strongest in those parts of the world with depleted ozone, have a two- to threefold increase in resveratrol production. That is why grapes from high-altitude vineyards such as those in Argentina, Sardinia, and some areas of Russia have among the highest concentrations.

Resveratrol itself is an off-white powder found in two forms, depending on the structure of the molecule. *Trans-resveratrol* is the more active form, preferred for use in supplements. It is relatively stable if protected from light, oxygen, and a high-pH environment. If exposed to light, however, it will rapidly convert to the less stable form and lose much of its biological effect. Dried red grape skins yield approximately 92 milligrams of resveratrol from 1 kilogram of grape skins, which is approximately a 1,000:1 ratio. This means that very large amounts of red grape skins are required to produce resveratrol.

Quercetin

Quercetin was found to be second only to resveratrol as a potent sirtuin-gene-activating xeno factor. In the polyphenol family, quercetin is considered a flavonol, one of the most active antioxidants of the polyphenols found in medicinal plants. In addition to stressed grapes and wine, foods rich in quercetin are apples, black and green tea, onions (particularly the outermost rings), citrus fruits, cherries, and various berries.

Many medicinal plants are believed to owe their biological activity to high quercetin content. Quercetin has known anti-inflammatory effects, and it helps to prevent cancer, prostatitis, heart disease, cataracts, allergies, bronchitis, and asthma. It also enhances the absorption of resveratrol and prolongs its effects.

Stability

It is now well established that the polyphenols found in red wine, red grape juice, and red grape skins, including resveratrol, are synergistic: that is, they act in concert to exert their biological effects. This adds to the stability of the mixture. The effectiveness of any nutraceutical or drug depends, among other things, on its stability. Exposure to light, high temperatures, and air is known to degrade the potency and effectiveness of xeno factors; therefore the extraction and manufacturing processes are critical to their ultimate effectiveness.

Approximately four years ago, an unpublished study from the Anti-aging Laboratory at Harvard University indicated that few available over-the-counter resveratrol-containing supplements possessed sirtuin activating properties. This situation may have improved along with further refinements in manufacturing and storage. Xi Zhao-Wilson, chief executive officer of BioMarker Pharmaceuticals, puts it this way: "As for the variability of different available preparations [of resveratrol], this is always an issue with respect to manufacturing and quality control associated with dietary supplements in general. It is 'buyer beware,' and one must find a high-quality source with a vested interest in providing consumers with the best available products and scientific evidence to back them up."

Absorption

Some of the most strident criticisms of the use of xeno factors and, in particular, resveratrol, focus on its absorption into the bloodstream and the actual bioavailability of the xeno factors. A brief discussion of how ingested substances enter the bloodstream can help us understand this issue. When these plant foods are ingested, they pass from the stomach into the intestines and then are transported by the blood to the liver. This transformation of foods into biologically active substances occurs through complex chemical pathways. For example, one major pathway leads either to activation or to deactivation of any drug we ingest. Another process links desirable molecules in the liver to ingested substances to allow for easier transport and delivery to the cells, and speeds the elimination of toxic substances through the kidneys or bile.

In the case of polyphenols, and, in particular, resveratrol and quercetin, sulfur and sugarlike molecules (metabolites) attach themselves to the xeno factors, so there is very little "free" resveratrol left to circulate in the blood. Because of this low resveratrol blood level, some scientists believed these xeno factors were of little benefit. In 2004 Thomas Walle and his colleagues at the Medical University of South Carolina gave human subjects both intravenous and oral resveratrol. They then measured the blood levels from the intestine and concluded that the absorption rate was very high. The amount of resveratrol in the blood, however, was very low. They did note a large accumulation of resveratrol in the cells lining the digestive tract and suggested that resveratrol may be an active cancer preventive in this organ as well as the liver. Despite the relatively low blood level, Dr. Walle and his team discovered that the resveratrol attached to sulfur and the sugarlike molecules could be found in the blood for a long time—up to 18.5 hours after a single dose.

Since xeno factors are therapeutic in so many diseases, Joseph Baur and David Sinclair concluded from Walle's results that "the undeniable in vivo efficacy of resveratrol, despite its low bioavailability [in blood levels] has led to speculation that its metabolites could retain some activity." Confirming studies on the resveratrol metabolites themselves demonstrate that they retain their ability to activate the SIRT1 enzyme and thereby reduce inflammation.

We also know that in various disease states such as cancer, inflammation, and diseases of the liver and intestine, an enzyme is produced that "unbinds" the sulfur and the sugar, making xeno factor available to those tissues that need it the most; this may explain their effectiveness in so many different diseases.

There is another observation often overlooked by those critical of the low blood levels of resveratrol and xeno factors. Several studies have now confirmed that quercetin inhibits the attachment of the sulfa molecule to resveratrol in the liver, thereby increasing the amount available in the bloodstream. Thus stressed plant polyphenols commonly found in red grapes not only are bioactive themselves but are synergistic in promoting health benefits. Optimal absorption and benefit appear to occur when resveratrol is included with other polyphenols like quercetin.

Safety

Since the report of the French paradox in 1992, there has been an explosion of scientific interest in red wine. When the polyphenols from the skin of the red wine grape responsible for the health-promoting effects are extracted and concentrated into the tablet equivalent of several hundred bottles of wine, the critical question becomes: is it safe?

The FDA's Center for Drug Evaluation and Research publishes guidelines for selecting the maximum recommended starting dose (MRSD) for clinical trials of new drug compounds. The first step is to establish that there are no observed adverse effects in test animals and/or people, a process that begins after the toxicity data have been analyzed. Although plant polyphenols are not drugs, they clearly are bioactive. Scientists who study natural food supplements are using techniques similar to those of the pharmaceutical industry to evaluate the potential health benefits of these plant polyphenols in animals and people.

Animal and Laboratory Studies

In 2002 the National Institute of Environmental Health Sciences commissioned a report entitled "Trans-resveratrol: Review of Toxicological Literature." This review of more than two hundred referenced scientific studies reported no adverse effects from resveratrol. Animal studies have used up to 300 milligrams per kilogram of weight a day of resveratrol, which would be equivalent to almost 1.5 grams (1,500 milligrams) per day for the average 170-pound male, and have shown no side effects. Much of the basic research on the effects of resveratrol has been performed on animal and human cells in test tubes with pure resveratrol concentrations that are often ten to one hundred times greater than the maximum concentrations observed in humans after oral consumption.

Resveratrol, like soy and many other natural substances, has a structure that is somewhat similar to the naturally occurring hormone estrogen. Because of this, some scientists have expressed concern that resveratrol may have some estrogen effect that could adversely influence breast tissue or abnormal cells like cancers. But resveratrol is about seven times *less* estrogen active than soy found in many foods.

Concern about estrogen effects arose from a 1997 study done by Dr. Barry Gehm at Northwestern University Medical School. He flooded breast cancer cells with pure resveratrol in a test tube and found that it stimulated the growth of estrogen-dependent breast cancer cells. Other studies have led to opposite findings, showing that resveratrol *stops* the growth of breast cancer cells. Additionally, the data from Gehm's study cannot be compared with the biological activity of orally administered resveratrol, because when resveratrol is ingested, it is broken down in the liver before reaching the bloodstream. In other words, after the passage through the liver, the concentration in the blood is reduced markedly when compared with applying unmetabolized "pure" resveratrol directly to cancer cells in a test tube. Additionally, the concentration of resveratrol used in the study was about ten times greater than even the most massive doses given to humans. Neither the purity nor the source was mentioned in his study, and extrapolation to the human condition is inappropriate.

On the other hand, many studies confirm the cancer-preventive potential of resveratrol. In fact, in a more recent study from the Laboratory of Biochemistry and Molecular Biology at Italy's University of Milan, Francesca Scarlatti and associates concluded that resveratrol inhibits breast cancer cells, resulting in their death. The most important thing to note here is that no animal study in which resveratrol was injected or fed to animals to treat tumors has shown a detrimental result. On the contrary, the majority of these studies have shown an impressive anticancer effect.

Human Studies

Human observations also confirm the safety of resveratrol and other polyphenols in highly concentrated forms. There are now several clinical studies funded by the NIH investigating the safety and therapeutic benefits of resveratrol as part of a series of large-scale cancer studies. As discussed in the chapter on cancer, in a joint study conducted by Dr. David Boocock at the University of Leicester in the U.K. and Dr. Dean Brenner at the University of Michigan Comprehensive Cancer Center, three different oral doses of resveratrol given to twenty-nine healthy volunteers were deemed safe. The study found no significant side effects and no evidence of toxicity.

The Sirtris pharmaceutical company in Cambridge, Massachusetts, is focused on developing drugs that activate sirtuin genes to prevent or treat diseases. Using a proprietary formulation of resveratrol, researchers there administered the product in doses ranging up to 5 grams per day to eighty-five healthy male subjects to evaluate safety, dose tolerability, and absorption. A few subjects developed diarrhea and vomiting, but otherwise there were no serious side effects of any kind; overall, these high doses were very well tolerated.

Resveratrol supplements have been sold for more than six years with no major side effects reported. Human clinical trials using from 500 to 5,000 milligrams of resveratrol have found these dosages to be safe. In fact, resveratrol supplements appear to be safer than alcoholic beverages, ibuprofen, and even aspirin. There are now multiple ongoing studies, particularly of resveratrol, funded by the National Institutes of Health and other government-sponsored research centers, evaluating its safety and efficacy. As of late 2008 I am aware of no research study reporting significant adverse side effects in humans taking resveratrol as a health supplement.

Finally, in the study of human memory and endurance, James Smoliga used the Australian extract, quercetin, and resveratrol in two experimental groups compared with a placebo group. Over the course

TABLE 5. FDA Guidelines to Calculate Animal-to-Human Equivalent Dosage

Animal	Amount Given	Human Equivalent Dose	Equivalent to 1-Liter Bottle of Wine (1–3 Milligrams)
Rat	80 milligrams per kilogram of weight	896	180 bottles
Rat	250 milligrams per kilogram of weight	2,800	560 bottles
Dog	2,000 grams per kilogram of weight	75,600	15,120 bottles
Mouse	22.4 milligrams per kilogram of weight	125 milligrams	25 bottles
Mouse	400 milligrams per kilogram of weight	2,240 grams	448 bottles

of three months, he found no evidence of side effects, intolerance, or toxicity in any of the ninety experimental subjects.

From the available toxicological literature in both animals and humans, the natural plant compounds of resveratrol and the polyphenols found in wine and concentrated in products like the Australian extract have a history of safe use and have shown no adverse side effects.

Since the 2002 NIH report, several hundred additional animal and laboratory studies have appeared in the literature evaluating treatment of various diseases as well as dosing and toxicity of resveratrol. Reports confirm the safety of these natural compounds in large doses.

Dosage

Here's a question I hear all the time: How much should I take? Although longer-term studies are needed in the search for longevity, many researchers are attempting to quantify the optimal dose to capture the potential clinical benefits of xeno factors. As scientist Xi Zhao-Wilson of BioMarker Pharmaceuticals puts it, "Extrapolation of an optimal dose from animal studies to humans is always more of an art than a science, and the appropriate studies still need to be done. Nevertheless, reasonable assumptions can be made, and there is even evidence that low doses may be effective for certain conditions."

It is helpful to begin our calculations by reviewing the amount of red wine (and polyphenols contained therein) that are necessary to stimulate the health benefits of the French paradox. Although table 6 lists only a few examples, there is a wide variation in the concentration of resveratrol. But in general, red wine has a significantly higher amount than other wines.

Additionally, the type of grape and the wine produced also influence the resveratrol amount. Pinot Noir wines generally have the highest levels, followed by Merlot, grenache, Cabernet Sauvignon, and tempranillo.

Given the chemicals used in most commercial vineyards to suppress the fungal stresses on grapes, which produce a lower resveratrol content, it is estimated that most wines contain 1 to 5 milligrams of

TABLE 6. Total Resveratrol Content of Wines and Grape Juice

Beverage	Total Resveratrol (Milligrams per Liter)	Total Resveratrol in a 5-Ounce Glass (Milligrams)
White wines (Spanish)	0.05–1.80	0.01–0.27
Rosé wines (Spanish)	0.43–3.52	0.06–0.53
Red wines (Spanish and French)	1.92–12.59	0.29–1.89
Red wines (global)	1.98–7.13	0.30–1.07
Red grape juice (Spanish)	1.14–8.69	0.17–1.30

resveratrol per liter. Although there are now several boutique wineries that claim higher amounts of resveratrol in their wines, if you were to consume two glasses (approximately 375 milliliters) a day, you would be ingesting, at most, approximately 1.5 milligrams of resveratrol. A similar amount of other unconcentrated polyphenols (or xeno factors) would also be consumed in those two glasses of wine. Even at this low level, these polyphenols do offer some health benefits (according to the French paradox), as well as protection against the toxic effects of alcohol in wine. Beyond two glasses, however, the additional alcohol nullifies the polyphenol's protective effect and increases the possibility of cirrhosis and brain damage.

It's instructive to look at the amounts given to live animals by the investigators at Harvard, in France, and recently at the University of Wisconsin to obtain the dramatic results they all reported. In the Harvard study, the amount given to mice that increased their survival, insulin sensitivity, and mitochondrial numbers, and improved their strength and endurance, translates into a human dose in the range of 150 to 200 milligrams per day. The Lagouge-Auwerx study used 400 milligrams per kilogram of body weight to obtain its dramatic zero weight gain on a high-calorie diet and its profound endurance and strength improvements. Compensating for the slower metabolic rate of humans versus mice and using FDA guidelines would change the

TABLE 7. Total Resveratrol Content of Selected Foods

Food	Serving	Total Resveratrol (Milligrams)
Peanuts (raw)	1 cup (146 grams)	0.01–0.26
Peanuts (boiled)	1 cup (180 grams)	0.32–1.28
Peanut butter	1 cup (258 grams)	0.04–0.13
Red grapes	1 cup (160 grams)	0.24–1.25

human equivalent dose to approximately 2,300 milligrams per day. In June 2008 fifteen scientists led by Drs. Richard Weindruch and Tomas Prolla from the University of Wisconsin reported their results with very low doses of resveratrol. They used 4 to 9 milligrams per kilogram of weight a day in mice and found that a low dose of dietary resveratrol partially mimics caloric restriction and slows aging in mice. They concluded: "Resveratrol, at doses that can be readily achieved in humans, fulfills the definition of a dietary compound that mimics some aspects of calorie restriction." Their human equivalent dose would be approximately 50 to 55 milligrams.

Therefore we have studies suggesting that resveratrol doses ranging from 50 to 200 milligrams could produce significant health benefits. Interestingly, Dr. Auwerx was quoted as saying that he took 40 milligrams per day, and many scientists in the Harvard lab self-administer approximately 200 milligrams per day or more. This is equivalent to drinking between forty and two hundred bottles of red wine per day!

The largest amounts in humans are being used experimentally. David Boocock is using a 5-gram dose (five thousand bottles of wine) to evaluate human tolerance, for a colon cancer study. Scientists at Sirtris Pharmaceuticals are investigating similar amounts in humans for possible treatment of cancer and diabetes.

Perhaps the most compelling information—even though it is anecdotal (that is, not based on a scientific study)—concerning the use of resveratrol supplements comes from a survey of Sirtris investors (or those interested in the company). This poll was conducted in February 2008, via web log, and revealed that 80 percent of those responding were taking resveratrol, and in the following amounts):

Not taking any: 19 percent
Up to 100 milligrams: 11 percent
Up to 200 milligrams: 20 percent
Up to 1,000 milligrams: 26 percent
Over 1,000 milligrams: 22 percent

Given the results of Sirtris's type 2 diabetes clinical trial, in which doses of 5,000 milligrams and 2,500 milligrams had no adverse effects, it is not surprising that those most knowledgeable about sirtuins are taking the highest doses. Resveratrol supplements now on the market contain anywhere from 8 to 500 milligrams per dose. As resveratrol continues to capture headlines, companies are clamoring to ride the rising commercial tide and produce new resveratrol formulations.

The final question is: should people consume xeno factors as supplements or just from foods? Many of the research scientists in this area themselves take supplements, thereby voting with their actions. This trend also speaks volumes about safety and potential health benefits. Again, Zhao-Wilson, a research scientist noted particularly for her work on the metabolic activities of resveratrol, considered the question and stated, "The properties associated with resveratrol appear to be largely protective—cardio-protective, anticancer, anti-inflammatory—and the current data suggest that most people can benefit from dietary supplementation with resveratrol obtained from a high-quality source." She further believes that it is generally safe when taken in conventional dosages.

Chapter 17

The Hows and Whys of Overweight

The doctor of the future will give no medicine but will interest his patients in the care of the human frame, and diet, and in the cause and prevention of disease.

—THOMAS EDISON

I believe that how we eat is an important determinant of how we feel and how we age. I also believe that food can function as medicine to influence a variety of common ailments.

—DR. ANDREW WEIL, *EATING WELL FOR OPTIMUM HEALTH*

No matter how much red wine or resveratrol you consume, a longer and healthier life—the goal to which I hope this book will contribute—requires a healthy lifestyle and dietary discretion. The reason is simple. Every major disease we've discussed—diabetes, cancer, heart disease, Alzheimer's—is either caused by or aggravated by excess weight. This is why we will explore the hows and whys of weight gain in this chapter, and then move on to discuss the Longevity Diet.

Maintaining a relatively normal weight may be essential to achieving good health and longevity, but as most of us know, this is much easier suggested than done.

- Approximately 60 percent of Americans are overweight or obese.
- Forty-one percent of Americans (approximately 120 million!) are currently trying to lose weight.

- Physicians believe that obesity is America's most severe health issue.
- Recent statistics show a dramatic rise (200 percent!) in the number of children hospitalized for type 2 diabetes.
- Excess weight is a direct cause of diabetes, heart disease, many cancers, stroke, arthritis, and depression.
- Supersized portions and lack of exercise are the greatest contributors to the problem.

The above facts are daily reminders of how fat we are becoming and the health consequences of the extra weight we carry. This is why the diet business has never been in better shape—unlike many of its customers. What's more, cunning promulgation of fear, stereotypes, and biases is a trademark of this industry motivated by the bottom line. In the United States alone, annual spending on diet products runs between $75 billion and $100 billion, more than the combined government budgets for health, education, and welfare!

There is a tremendous amount of social pressure to diet in our American culture. A slim shape is equated with health, success, and even character. Overweight people are reminded by a barrage of media to blame themselves for their failed weight-loss programs. All too often, our culture focuses on lack of "willpower" as the reason for obesity. Among women it is almost a social requirement to be on a "lose-weight-fast" program or to belong to a diet center. And although it's also important socially to belong to a local health club, most members are just that: members, not participants.

Two recent studies found that weight discrimination might be as common as racial bias. Overweight individuals are fired, denied jobs or promotions, and discriminated against through insults, abuse, and harassment by others. A research survey of more than two thousand adults reported that discrimination based on weight has increased 66 percent in the past decade, according to one study in the journal *Obesity*. Those who are severely overweight feel they are treated the worst, particularly women, nearly half of whom perceive discrimination due to their appearance.

In my neurosurgical practice, which is strongly oriented toward patients with spinal and disk problems, 70 percent of my patients over fifty-five are overweight or obese. Because of my own genetic predisposition to being overweight, I have been keenly interested in the diet "du jour," not only for my patients but also for me. In fact, to better understand the potential impact of a diet based on the principles of xenohormesis, I reviewed dozens of separate diets (see the list below) from A to Z, from Atkins to Zone.

Partial List of Available Weight-Loss Diets

100-Mile diet
Abs diet
Atkins diet
Banta diet
Best Bet diet
Blood Type diet
Body for Life
Breatharian diet
Buddhist diet
Cabbage soup diet
Calorie restriction
Cambridge diet
Candida control diet
Cretan diet
Detox diet
Diabetic diet
Diet Smart Plan
Dietary Approaches to Stop Hypertension (DASH) diet
Dr. Hay diet
eDiets
Fat Resistance diet
Fat Smash diet
Feingold diet
Fit for Life diet

Flexitarian diet

Food Combining diet

Fruitarian diet

Gerson diet

Gluten-free, Casein-free diet

Glycemic Index diet

Graham diet

Grapefruit diet

Hacker's diet

Halal diet

Hallelujah diet

High-protein diet

Hunza diet

Jenny Craig program

Joel Fuhrman diet

Junk Food diet

Kosher diet

Lacto-vegetarianism

Lean for Life

Liquitarian diet

Living Foods diet

Low-carbohydrate diet

Low-protein diet

Macrobiotic diet

Master Cleanse

Mediterranean diet

Montignac diet

Natural Foods diet

Natural Hygiene diet

Negative Calorie diet

No-grain diet

Okinawa diet

Optimal diet

Organic Food diet

Ornish diet

Ovo-lacto-vegetarian diet

Paleolithic diet

Perricone diet

Pescetarian diet

PersonalDiets

Plant-based diet

Pollotarian diet

Pritikin diet

Rastafarian diet

Raw Foodism

Rice diet/Duke University diet

Scarsdale diet

Sex diet

Shangri-La diet

Slimming World diet

South Beach diet

Sonoma diet

Sugar Busters

T-Factor diet

Total Wellbeing diet

Vegan diet

Vegetarian diet

Warrior diet

Weigh Down diet

Weight Watchers

Zone diet

Each diet was, of course, accompanied by the requisite book, an often meteoric best seller full of scientific explanations that sounded compelling, at least at first. These diets usually are promoted as quick, *permanent* cures for obesity. But the statistics on permanence are abysmal. Recent medical surveys and research indicate that 95 percent of all dieters fail to lose a significant amount of weight or fail to maintain that weight loss over five years. Sadly, a third of all dieters actually *gain* weight!

The Hows of Excess Weight

Many theories are offered to explain the obesity epidemic, including genetic predisposition, abnormality in the hunger and satiety centers of the brain, abnormal absorption of nutrients from the intestine, hormonal abnormalities of the thyroid, and failures in the regulation of insulin. Socioeconomics may also play a part. The food choices of women in supermarket checkout lines who cash in food stamps show an emphasis on quantity over quality, leading to an overabundance of snacks and sweets.

Obesity in parents increases the likelihood of obesity in children, thanks to both genetic and environmental factors. In July 2007 a landmark research study published in the prestigious *New England Journal of Medicine* showed that obesity is socially contagious—that people's obesity can significantly increase the risk of obesity among their friends, siblings, or spouses. Thinness was also found to be contagious: if a person slims down, those around him or her are more likely to lose weight as well.

Finally, and perhaps most important, psychological factors have a powerful effect on obesity. We overeat in search of relief from stress, pain, depression, anxiety, and low self-esteem. We overeat because we are out of balance emotionally. In May 2008 *USA Today* concluded its fifth annual weight-loss challenge. Headlines read, "Dieters Navigate Tides of Emotion" and "Successful Dieters Distinguish Hunger from Emotions." Psychologists and nutrition experts alike observe that emotional eating is rampant in this country.

Although any and all of these factors may be influential, the basic cause of the obesity epidemic is excessive caloric intake and an inadequate expenditure of energy. Simply put, we eat way too much and exercise way too little.

In addition, Americans have developed an incredible sweet tooth. According to the *Harvard Health Letter,* in 2006 we consumed approximately one hundred pounds of sweeteners per person. One of these sweeteners, high-fructose corn syrup, may be one of the worst culprits in the U.S. diet. Researchers are coming to believe that our bodies process the sugar in high-fructose corn syrup differently from cane or beet sugar, and that this difference affects the way our metabolic-regulating hormones function. It also forces the liver to kick more fat out into the bloodstream. The end result is that our bodies get tricked into wanting to eat more while at the same time storing more fat!

Another danger zone is beverages. Marketers of sports beverages and juice drinks, another multibillion-dollar industry, promote the "healthful" benefits of these beverages, but one problem is that people don't cut back on their overall caloric intake to offset the extra calories from such products. Harvard researchers recently reported that women who drank one or more fructose-sweetened soft drinks per day were 83 percent more likely to develop type 2 diabetes than women who drank less than one a month. Not surprisingly, they were also likely to gain more weight.

We Americans are also remarkably sedentary. Fewer and fewer of us earn our livelihoods through physical labor, and with the advent of television and computers, we've taken to sitting during most of our nonwork time. Our bodies, which were built for nearly constant physical activity, are lucky now if we use them to do something physical two or three times a week. Many of us don't exercise at all.

Interestingly, Dr. Keith Ayoob, who works with overweight patients at the Albert Einstein College of Medicine in New York City, states, "I need to help the patients balance not just their diet, but their lifestyle. Food shouldn't be your only source of fun," he says. In chapter 18 I outline a formula for doing just that: achieving balance, in your diet and in your life.

Cravings and the Brain—The Whys

Excess calories and insufficient exercise are a plausible explanation for the "how" of the obesity epidemic. But the "why" is even more intriguing to me. Why do 90 percent to 95 percent of people fail on a diet plan? The "uncontrollable" urge to eat—often greater on a diet—reminds me of a twenty-two-year-old motorcycle head injury victim whom I cared for several years ago. Traveling at about sixty miles an hour, he struck a bridge abutment and was brought comatose to the hospital. So severe was his brain injury that he was being considered as an organ donor. A CT scan showed major damage to his temporal lobes (located just inside the skull, by the ear). To everyone's surprise, he made an amazing recovery and was discharged to a rehabilitation center.

The next time I saw him was six months later. He came to my office accompanied by his loving but exhausted wife. The young man's demeanor was curious, a combination of flat affect and carefree unconcern. His wife asked if she could speak to me alone and then described his incredible personality change. This previously thin, controlled, fastidious graduate student in accounting had developed a ravenous appetite and was markedly obese. He had become an eating machine. He had also developed an almost insatiable sexual appetite. When his wife could no longer satisfy his needs for sex three to five times per day, he became a frequent visitor to houses of ill repute in the Pittsburgh area. Her question to me was, "Doctor, why? What has happened to him?"

Her question triggered my memory of a lecture by Dr. Paul Bucy, professor of neurosurgery at Northwestern University, many years earlier. Dr. Bucy was a visiting professor at Indiana University when I was the chief neurosurgical resident there, and I had the good fortune to meet this icon of neurosurgery and attend his lecture on the activity of the temporal lobes of the brain. He described how he and his associate Heinrich Klüver, a German neuroscientist, were evaluating injuries to temporal lobes in monkeys when they found the same striking behavioral changes I later saw in my patient: an insatiable appetite with an excessive oral fixation, hypersexuality, and blunted emotional responses. Subsequently, this syndrome, or constellation of symptoms, was named Klüver-Bucy syndrome.

Fast-forward to April 2007, and we find a report in the *Journal of the American Medical Association*: "Brain Scans, Genes Provide Addiction Clues." It has long been recognized that food can be addictive. In another *JAMA* article that same month, Nora D. Volkow, MD, director of the National Institute on Drug Abuse, described using modern neuroimaging of the brain to confirm that cravings for recreational drugs share a similar brain mechanism with cravings for food. In obese people, food functions like a drug! Because of ongoing imbalances in hormonal and/or emotional areas, overweight individuals tend to continually self-medicate to get another "fix" (usually from carbohydrates and fats) to maintain the feel-good feeling. This unbalanced diet contributes even further to an unbalanced emotional and physical lifestyle, leading us to join the 60 percent of overweight Americans. So although genetics, hormonal balances, and intestinal absorption problems may well account for some cases of obesity, neurochemically mediated brain responses to physical and emotional imbalance are perhaps the major reason for the obesity epidemic.

The Role of Inflammation in Obesity

The "pleasure center" of the brain, called the nucleus accumbens, processes our responses to food, drugs, and other sources of pleasure like sex and even video games. When it is functioning normally, the nucleus accumbens is an integral, positive part of our emotional life. When hijacked by food addiction, it becomes detrimental. This is not unlike the process of inflammation: when functioning normally, it protects us from damage of all kinds; if it runs amok, it contributes to all the diseases we have been discussing: diabetes, cancer, heart disease, stroke, arthritis, Parkinson's, and Alzheimer's.

Most inflammation, as we know it, is visible. When we get a bee sting, a splinter in a finger, or a sprained ankle, we experience redness, swelling, pain, and heat. Hidden inflammation, on the other hand— inflammation inside our bodies—has now been recognized as a missing link in the obesity epidemic. In chapter 10's discussion of diabetes, we explored the dangers of chronically elevated levels of insulin as well as high blood sugar. Excess blood sugar increases the body's fat, which itself is now recognized as a source of factors that lead to chronic inflammation.

A certain amount of fat is necessary for health and wellness. This level is usually regulated by a hormone called leptin, which, interestingly, is produced by the fat tissue itself. As we add more and more fat tissue to our bodies, leptin is released. In healthy people, leptin suppresses appetite and speeds up metabolism, reducing feelings of hunger while the body is burning more calories and losing excess fat. But chronic inflammation impairs the brain's ability to receive leptin's message. Like insulin resistance, which we discussed in connection with diabetes, this situation is called leptin resistance. With leptin resistance, fat accumulates.

What are the most important factors contributing to inflammation and, secondarily, to overweight? Stress, sugar, trans fats, toxins in our food and environment, infections, overall poor nutrition, and lack of exercise. Foods with a high glycemic index—which rates how quickly a carbohydrate breaks down into sugar—are particularly strong triggers of inflammation. These foods contribute to insulin resistance, which results in increased body fat storage.

The mind-body contribution to inflammation and weight gain is best exemplified by our response to stress. Mild to moderate short-term stress is good for both, whereas prolonged, chronic distress can be fatal.

The body responds to stress in our daily lives by releasing from the adrenal glands a hormone called cortisol. Cortisol is involved in the metabolism of carbohydrate, fat, and protein, and in the body's immune response, and it is also helpful as an anti-inflammatory. If elevated by stress for prolonged periods, however, it has a powerful destructive effect on the body. Cortisol suppresses the immune system. It increases our appetite, and the excess calories plus cortisol lead us to accumulate fat, particularly in the abdominal region. This so-called central obesity leads to many of the diseases already discussed: heart disease, diabetes, strokes, and more. Stress management, therefore, is a central part of any effective weight-loss program.

In all of the diseases that we have discussed, including obesity, the common theme is gene activation. The primary contributors to weight gain and the epidemic of obesity-related diseases are physical factors such as hormonal abnormalities; psychological factors dealing with stress, cravings, and addictions; and unlimited access to high-calorie, high-fat food products. Each of these acts as a "medicine," according to

Dr. Andrew Weil, "to influence a variety of common ailments or to contribute to them through genetic factors." The next part of the book provides concrete suggestions, given our present level of understanding, for what each of us can do to activate genes that counter the negative effects we've just mentioned, and to trigger biochemicals that actively contribute to our health and longevity.

Part IV

Unlocking the Genetic Secrets to Living Healthier and Longer

Chapter 18

What's a Person to Do?

One can never put one's foot into the same river twice.

—HERACLEITUS, 450 BC

Resveratrol-like drugs could have as big an impact as antibiotics in the twentieth century, and it's just around the corner.

—DAVID SINCLAIR, WORLD SCIENCE FESTIVAL, 2008

Dramatic new scientific discoveries have unlocked the genetic secrets to a longer and healthier life. As so often happens with great discoveries, the answers turn out to be based on an incredibly simple idea: by ingesting natural plant molecules with which we have coexisted for millions of years, we can switch genes on and off to benefit from their anti-inflammatory, anticancer, antibacterial, and blood sugar–normalizing effects—and live longer!

Although most research to date has focused on resveratrol as the primary gene activating compound, with the greatest number of health benefits, thousands of other polyphenol compounds found in plants and plant products have similar health benefits. In fact, many scientists believe it is a combination of these polyphenols found in plants themselves—and not just a single ingredient—that provides the most stable source of healthy gene activating molecules. This is why a daily glass or two of red wine, which contains not just resveratrol but a combination of more than five hundred other polyphenols, provides such scientifically well-documented health benefits.

The resveratrol story is still evolving rapidly. After reviewing thousands of medical articles, books, and scientific studies and visiting David Sinclair's mouse lab at Harvard Medical School, I believe that we are already beginning to see a tidal wave in the world of gene activating food additives and supplements. As more and more are discovered, they will be added to the foods we eat as supplements, until one day they will be as common as folic acid is now in prenatal vitamins, preventing devastating birth defects. The products available and recommended today may be substantially increased in number or modified in other ways over the next few years—or even months—on the basis of results of ongoing scientific laboratory and human studies.

Recognizing this, we still have remarkable opportunities to make the most of the scientific discoveries to date. What should you do? In accordance with the principles that I have outlined in these pages, there are four ways you can access the secrets of genetics to live longer and healthier.

1. Eat and drink natural foods with the highest polyphenol antioxidant content, such as red wine, grape juice, green tea, dark chocolate, and apples.
2. Take supplements containing superconcentrated polyphenol and resveratrol from natural sources.
3. Take resveratrol, with or without additional polyphenols, as a dietary supplement.
4. Use a prescription resveratrol-like drug.

Let's look at each of these individually.

1. Polyphenols and Health

We have discussed polyphenols' role in preventing inflammation and possibly cancer, heart attacks, and strokes as well. The earliest recorded use of polyphenols to cure disease dates back to the North America of the French explorer Jacques Cartier in 1534. He and his crew were near death when they were revived by a Native American concoction of pine bark and needles that was extremely rich in a particular polyphenol called procyanidin. This potent antioxidant, now marketed as pycnogenol for its effect on the heart and blood vessels, is part of the same family of polyphenols that provide amazing health benefits and are found in red wine, chocolate, blueberries, cranberries, and more. It too is produced by plants to defend themselves against funguses, toxins, and environmental stresses such as excessive heat or cold, extremes in humidity, and the sun's ultraviolet rays.

Let's take a closer look at the remarkable health benefits of a few of the most popular foods with the highest resveratrol-antioxidant content.

Drink Wine!

Wine making dates back to at least 5500 BC. Seeds used for fermentation have been found in excavated Bronze Age dwellings near the Caspian Sea in southwestern Asia. Wine consumption played an important role in ancient Egyptian ceremonial life three thousand years ago. The ancient Greeks referred to wine as the nectar of the gods, knowing that *nectar* means "that which overcomes death." How appropriate that 2,500 years after the golden age of Greece we should be discussing the role of resveratrol in enhanced longevity.

Nearly all of the wine made in the world comes from one species of grape: the *Vitis vinifera*. Although there are as many as four thousand varieties of grapes, only about a dozen are frequently used for wine making. The chief varieties include Chardonnay, Riesling, Cabernet Sauvignon, Pinot Noir, sauvignon blanc, Gewürztraminer, and Merlot, among others. It is the high sugar content of the *Vitis vinifera,* when ripe, that allows it to produce wine.

As previously discussed, grapes—in particular, red wine grapes—are the single greatest source of resveratrol in our diet. Interestingly, new research shows that dark chocolate is the second greatest source for many people. (Other sources are listed in table 2 on page 49.) The qualities of the soil, type of grape, altitude, climate, UV radiation, fungal infection, and the specific process of wine making used all contribute to the amount of resveratrol and other gene activating compounds in the wine. During the fermentation process, sugars in the grapes are converted into alcohol and carbon dioxide. In the case of red wines, the longer the skins, seeds, and pulp are fermented together, the higher the resveratrol and polyphenol content of the wine.

Health Benefits of Red Wine

Hundreds of scientific studies indicate that no more than two glasses of red wine per day for a man and one glass for a woman may provide the following health benefits:

- Reduces the risk of death from nearly all causes: Studies from France, the U.K., Finland, and Denmark indicate that moderate consumption of wine is more beneficial than beer or spirits in promoting longevity.
- Helps prevent coronary heart disease by reducing low-density lipoprotein (LDL) cholesterol and boosting high-density lipoprotein (HDL) cholesterol.
- Produces anticlotting action that prevents the formation of life-threatening blood clots.
- Prevents hardening of the arteries by promoting the formation of nitric oxide, the key relaxing factor for vascular tone.
- Can lower blood pressure in people with hypertension.
- Decreases the risk of kidney stone formation.
- Decreases the risk of Alzheimer's disease.
- Decreases the harmful effects of smoking on the lining of the blood vessels.

Is It the Resveratrol, the Alcohol, or the Other Polyphenols? Although red wines from Pinot Noir, Merlot, grenache, Cabernet Sauvignon, and tempranillo grapes have the highest resveratrol content, the total amount in a bottle of wine is still relatively low. Depending on the grape type, it may range from minimal to 40 milligrams per liter.

Most wines contain between 1 and 5 milligrams of resveratrol per liter. Chemicals now used in most commercial vineyards to suppress the fungal stresses on grapes result in a lower resveratrol content. However, there are several boutique wineries that use special resveratrol activating techniques to boost the amount of resveratrol in their wines. But by consuming approximately two average-sized glasses of red wine a day, we would still consume no more than 10 milligrams of resveratrol.

When we look at the laboratory studies conducted by Sinclair, Lagouge, and their colleagues, we see that to obtain the same kinds of results in humans that they did in animals would require consuming 65 to 1,150 liter bottles of red wine per day! Still, we know that the French paradox does occur in humans, thanks to our consumption of red wine. Therefore the alcohol and/or other polyphenols in two glasses of red wine must have extremely beneficial properties. In fact, in a bottle of red wine, the total procyanidin/polyphenol content is 1 to 2 grams per liter, or about one thousand times more than the amount of resveratrol in that same liter bottle. This is why wine is referred to as a polyphenol cocktail.

It is known that alcohol alone from beer, spirits, and white wine may contribute to heart health benefits when taken in low to moderate amounts. But the health benefits of alcohol alone are not commensurate with those provided by the hundreds of other polyphenols in red wine, particularly in increasing length of life. Furthermore, quercetin, fisetin, and other polyphenols in red wine improve the absorption of resveratrol, giving it a biological impact far beyond its modest quantity.

With such health benefits, should doctors be prescribing wine for their patients? "Good wine," wrote William Shakespeare, "is a good familiar creature if it be well used." Many physicians now believe that the current data are so strong that it is incumbent upon them to inquire into the drinking habits of their patients and make them aware of the health benefits of moderate red wine consumption, provided there are no medical reasons that would contradict this advice. Others believe that there is insufficient information to encourage patients who do not drink wine to start. The potential risk of addiction, of liver disease due to excessive consumption (to reduce liver damage, it is best to drink red wine with meals), and of increased accident rates are all cautions to be considered. This is clearly a situation in which a little is good, but a lot may be extremely harmful. Paracelsus (1493–1541), a Swiss physician and chemist, said it best: "Wine is a food, a medicine, and a poison; it's just a question of dose."

Drink Grape Juice

Non–wine drinkers, take heart! You too may benefit from health-promoting, gene activating polyphenol compounds found in nonalcoholic red grape juice. In the early 1990s, when resveratrol was thought to be the active ingredient responsible for the French paradox, non–wine drinkers began to wonder if they could obtain similar benefits from drinking grape juice. Dr. Leroy Creasy, a professor at Cornell University, researched the question. He found that the polyphenol was as high and at times higher in grape juice, particularly juice from the Finger Lakes region of upper New York State. He later concluded that this was due to the cool, damp climate there that allowed fungi to attack local grapes. Since that time, many studies have demonstrated the health benefits of pure red grape juice from Concord and muscadine grapes, which are similar to the healthful effects of red wine.

A 2004 clinical study showed lowered blood pressure for men and women who drank two servings of grape juice a day. Other studies have found that grape juice reduces platelet stickiness, the tendency for blood to clot in patients with hardening of the arteries. Still other studies have demonstrated that grape juice can reduce the oxidation of LDL cholesterol and improve elasticity of arteries, much the same way that red wine does. All of this means that grape juice itself is protective, particularly against heart attacks and strokes.

More recently, laboratory studies indicate that red grape juice suppresses the growth of tumors in the initiation stage in breast cancer cells. It has also shown a preventive effect in the development of tumors in the prostate, as well as slowing the first stage of development of other cancers. Scientists at Tufts University have discovered that grape juice can improve memory and coordination: laboratory animals given grape juice were better able to navigate mazes and had better memory retention. So in addition to its antioxidant effect, grape juice may protect and facilitate brain cell function directly.

Red and dark-purple grapes consumed with the skins are also good sources of vitamins C, B_1, and B_6, plus potassium and fiber. But Concord and muscadine red grape juice is a more concentrated source of antioxidants and plant nutrients than grapes alone. Ninety percent of the nutrient benefit of the grape is in the skin and seeds, which are the two elements of the fruit often discarded when grapes are eaten fresh. In the process of making grape juice, however, the skin and seeds stay mixed with the pulp, or flesh, for an extended period of time. This allows powerful flavonoids and other polyphenols to seep into the juice.

One concern about commercially available processed red grape juice is that most grape juice is pasteurized using high heat, and this process can reduce or even inactivate polyphenols such as resveratrol. Additionally, most processed red grape juice products have sugars and preservatives added, and studies of these products often show resveratrol bound to a sugar molecule; the biological action of this form of resveratrol is believed to be reduced compared with that of the unbound trans-resveratrol found in larger amounts in red wine and in red grape skins themselves.

Raisins, which are dried grapes, are not a good source of plant nutrients. Resveratrol and other polyphenols are destroyed by the exposure to light and the oxidation that occur when raisins are dried in the air.

So how much red grape juice should one drink daily? A serving of one or two 4- to 8-ounce glasses is suggested for optimal cardiovascular and health benefits. Because each serving contains a significant amount of natural sugars—up to 150 calories in 8 ounces—it should be used not as a replacement for water but as a replacement for flavored beverages and sodas, and as a complement to meals. Mixing it with seltzer or soda water as a spritzer makes for a refreshing soft-drink substitute.

Drink Green Tea

Tea is the most widely consumed beverage in the world, second only to water. Worldwide, per capita consumption is approximately 40 liters per year. Black tea is preferred in the Western world, and in the United States iced black tea makes up 80 percent of tea consumption. In Asian countries, green tea is the drink of choice. Green tea consumption is thought to be responsible for the so-called Asian paradox, much the way that polyphenols and red wine are responsible for the French paradox.

Cigarette consumption in Asia is the highest in the world. It is well known that smoking leads to heart attacks, strokes, peripheral vascular disease, and cancer. Paradoxically, however, Japan and other Asian countries are among the lowest in the incidence of arteriosclerosis and lung cancer. In fact, it has been shown in several studies that the lowest risk is found in people who drink approximately 1.2 liters of green tea daily.

The Chinese have known of the medicinal benefits of green tea for at least four thousand years. Just as grapes and wine were spread throughout the world initially by the Phoenicians and later by other traders, tea was introduced to countries worldwide by tradesmen and travelers. The health benefits of green tea border on the unbelievable and are very similar to those described for resveratrol and red wine. The secret of green tea is that it is extremely rich in catechin polyphenols, the same catechins found coating the seeds of grapes and in wine.

The tea plant itself has the scientific name *Camellia sinensis.* Although it is native to China, it has spread to and is now cultivated in many countries across the world, predominantly in the tropical and subtropical zones. Black, green, oolong, and white tea are all prepared from the same leaves. The difference is in the harvesting, drying, fermentation, and roasting. Black tea roasting takes place after the harvested leaves are crushed and undergo browning (also called fermentation or oxidation). Oolong tea is allowed to undergo moderate drying and fermentation. Green tea is created when the tea leaves are steamed or heated immediately after harvesting. White tea is made from young tea buds and does not undergo fermentation. The fermentation and oxidation process naturally reduces the polyphenol content of black tea. Green tea and white tea have the highest concentrations of the active catechins because they do not go through this process. Therefore they are the best dietary source of this compound. Catechins represent 80 percent of polyphenol flavonoids in green tea, whereas in black tea they represent approximately 20 percent to 30 percent.

There are now thousands of scientific articles detailing the wealth of health benefits provided by catechins found in green tea.

- Antioxidative and antiaging effects: The catechins found in tea are twenty-five to one hundred times as potent as vitamins C and E. One cup of green tea provides more antioxidant activity than a serving of broccoli, spinach, carrots, or strawberries. This activity reduces the damaging effects of free radicals.
- Anticlotting effect: Green tea catechins act on blood platelets to prevent stickiness and clotting, reducing the number of strokes and heart attacks.
- Antiviral and cold prevention effects: Green tea catechins attach themselves firmly to the surface of the flu virus and prevent it from infecting the human oral and nasal mucous membranes. Red wine and tea also protect against hepatitis C.
- Control of high blood pressure: Green tea catechins suppress the enzyme that contracts blood vessels, easing high blood pressure.
- Cancer prevention: Catechins in green tea interfere with cancer development in all three stages.
- Green tea catechins control cholesterol by blocking enzymes in the intestine that contribute to the absorption of cholesterol. They suppress LDL and elevate HDL.
- They control high blood sugar levels by suppressing the enzymes that break down sugar into glucose.
- They maintain healthy intestinal flora by decreasing the number of harmful bacteria and fostering the growth of "good" bacteria such as bifidobacteria.

- They contribute to weight loss: Together with the caffeine in tea, catechins accelerate the burning of fat. Men given a combination of caffeine and green tea extract burned more calories and lost more weight than those given only caffeine or a placebo.
- They prevent bad breath: Catechins neutralize unpleasant oral odors by reducing oral bacteria.
- They prevent tooth decay: Catechins have a strong antibacterial effect and prevent the buildup of dental plaque.
- They inhibit osteoarthritis: Studies using human cartilage cells demonstrated that a catechin known as *ECGC* protects against in-flammatory degeneration and arthritis.

There are several additional points to keep in mind. To obtain these dramatic health benefits from green tea, relatively large amounts must be consumed. A minimum of three to ten cups a day is recommended. Larger amounts, up to ten cups a day, have been used for cancer prevention, and in Japan these are supplemented with additional green tea tablets for the treatment of cancer. Also, not all green tea is equal in its content of catechins. Premium green teas contain at least 100 milligrams of the catechin EGCG, whereas some green tea bags from commercial food giants can contain one-third or even less. Brewing is a major factor, too. Unless you are drinking a fusion, in which the green tea is already dissolved in water, the tea bag should be placed into boiling water for approximately three minutes to get the maximal diffusion of polyphenols.

Caffeine content also is a factor. Green tea usually contains about 20 percent of the caffeine found in a cup of regular coffee. High consumption may cause agitation, anxiety, and irritability in those susceptible to caffeine.

Lemon and milk are frequent additives to various teas. The citric acid in lemons appears to enhance the absorbability of the catechins in green tea. Milk, on the other hand, may negate some of the health benefits, particularly in black tea. (The casein proteins in milk are thought to adhere to the catechins and offset some of their health benefits.) One researcher suggested that the reason that the British, who are passionate about tea, have failed to make as much headway against cardiovascular disease as the French with their red wine and the Asians with their green tea is their penchant for adding milk to their tea.

Despite extremely high consumption in some countries, the only negative effect reported from drinking green tea is insomnia secondary to the caffeine content. These observations parallel the absence of side effects seen in similar studies using resveratrol.

Eat Dark Chocolate

What possible connection could dark chocolate have with resveratrol, red wine, and green tea? Polyphenols. Dark chocolate is made from seeds from the cocoa tree. More than two thousand years ago, Aztec and Mayan Indians were grinding cacao seeds to make a spicy, bitter chocolate drink. In the 1500s, when Spanish conquistadors brought the cacao seeds back to Spain, sweeteners were added. Because of the great expense of importing it back to Europe, this chocolate drink was enjoyed primarily by royalty or high-ranking members of the church. Its delicious taste and its recognized nutritional and restorative properties led it to be called "the food of the gods," much as in Homeric times wine was called "the nectar of the gods."

Modern chemistry has discovered powerful polyphenols in cocoa seeds. In fact, scientists in Belgium recently identified trans-resveratrol in dark chocolate and cocoa liquor extracts, which also contain catechins similar to those in green tea and procyanidins found in red wine. Laboratory studies and hundreds of human clinical trials using dark chocolate as a source of concentrated flavonols, a specific kind of polyphenol, have shown effects similar to those of wine and green tea. These include the following:

• Acts as a powerful antioxidant: 47 percent of Americans eat chocolate at least once per week, making it the third-highest daily source of antioxidants in the U.S. diet.

- Reduces atherosclerosis: contributes to an overall reduction in heart attacks; lowers cholesterol, LDL cholesterol, and triglycerides; and raises HDL cholesterol.
- Reduces blood clotting: affects platelet stickiness, particularly when used in combination with aspirin.
- Improves blood flow: increases nitric oxide to dilate blood vessels.
- Acts as an antihypertensive: a German study showed that those who ate 3.5 ounces of dark chocolate products daily for two weeks lowered their risk of heart attack and stroke by 10 percent to 20 percent.
- Positively affects blood sugar: enhances the effect of insulin and sugar utilization.
- Is good for the skin: researchers in Germany discovered that women who drank an antioxidant-rich hot chocolate for three months developed smoother, better-hydrated skin that was less vulnerable to sunburn.
- Enhances mood and may function as an antidepressant.

Again, it seems almost too good to be true that something so delicious can have such remarkable health benefits. Indeed, there are several cautions. Most commercially available cocoa-based beverages and chocolates contain few if any flavonols, owing to food-processing techniques. As with wine and tea, the origin, postharvest handling, and processing of the flavonol-laden cocoa bean determine its ultimate health benefits.

After seeds are collected from the cocoa pods, they are allowed to ferment for a period of time that may cover several days prior to drying, packaging, and shipping. The longer the fermentation period, the lower the flavonol content. Additional loss of flavonol occurs after the bulk cocoa is received by food manufacturers and roasted to develop flavor. Cocoa flavonols are very heat sensitive, so this process further reduces their beneficial effects. To counter the acidity produced by the cocoa flavonols, an alkalizing process called "dutching" is used, which further reduces the flavonol concentration. Finally, milk may be added to the chocolate.

The dark chocolate that provides significant health benefits is, therefore, a nonsweetened or minimally sweetened chocolate with little or no added milk and a cocoa content of at least 70 percent. The most commonly eaten milk chocolate is a highly sweetened alkalized chocolate with added milk powder or condensed milk and reduced cocoa content, which has very little in the way of flavonol value.

One health concern raised by chocolate consumption relates to its high fat content. However, research has shown that provided the total fat and calorie intake does not exceed recommended levels, dark chocolate does not represent an increased risk to health.

Unfortunately, chocolate manufacturers rarely label their products for flavonol content. Sometimes flavonols, which are somewhat bitter, are removed from darkened cocoa solids, so that even dark chocolate may have little or no flavonols and thus minimal health benefits. As a health-conscious consumer, what should you do? My approach is to select only high-quality chocolate with at least 70 percent cocoa that is unsweetened or slightly sweetened and comes in convenient bite-sized squares. One serving of natural, unsweetened cocoa powder (5 grams) or two or three dark chocolate squares will provide an amount of antioxidant that is higher even than that in blueberries and cranberries on a dry weight basis.

How much is enough? In an article in the *Journal of the American Medical Association* in August 2007, Dr. Dirk Taubert and his associates at the University of Cologne in Germany attempted to answer this question with regard to blood pressure. They found that a small amount—30 calories per day of dark chocolate—was effective in "efficiently reducing blood pressure." That is roughly the number of calories found in *one* Hershey's Kiss (unfortunately, though, those are milk chocolate). The researchers concluded that the blood pressure reduction from this amount of dark chocolate would reduce the relative risk of dying from a stroke by 8 percent, and from coronary artery disease by 5 percent.

An added bonus from dark chocolate comes from the mood-altering chemicals contained in the chocolate, which include serotonin, endorphins, and phenylethylamine. The brain releases these chemicals to beat the blues and promote a feeling of well-being. Ancient cultures considered chocolate an aphrodisiac.

Omega-3 fatty acids (fish oil) have demonstrated similar anti-inflammatory and mood-elevating effects. Perhaps a combination of dark chocolate, omega-3s, and a glass or two of red wine may provide all the mood stabilization and health benefits we need! It would certainly take us a big step in the right direction.

Probiotics are healthy bacteria that studies have shown work in our intestines to protect against infections, prevent some tumors, help recolonize the intestinal tract after the use of antibiotics, and strengthen our immune system. In fact a new "sweet" supplement containing probiotics has recently become available. I take it daily. It is an organic dark chocolate containing over one billion colonies of probiotics. The dark chocolate, itself a powerful antioxidant, prevents the breakdown of the bacteria enabling them to reach the intestine where they perform their beneficial functions. The use of probiotics has markedly increased over the past five to ten years, and next to omega-3 fish oil is the fastest-growing supplement.

An Apple a Day Does Keep the Doctor Away!

Professor Gazi Yasargil, acknowledged by his peers as *the* neurosurgeon of the twentieth century, still performs intricate brain surgery at age seventy-eight with the same skills he possessed forty years earlier. When I visited him in Zurich, Switzerland, prior to his relocation to the United States, I was astounded by his stamina, his incredibly brilliant mind, and his technical brilliance. After watching him work sixteen hours a day, I asked him his secret. Was it exercise? A new, unreleased European dietary supplement? Genetics? "No," he responded. "Apples!" He informed me that he ate two or three large apples every day. He had no problems with weight control, rarely developed colds or other illnesses, and still had the energy of a forty- or fifty-year-old, with no signs of mental or physical deterioration.

I subsequently looked into the health benefits of apples and discovered that they are also high in procyanidin content and contain a unique polyphenol, phloridzin. Again I was struck by the many scientific papers substantiating the health benefits of an apple a day:

- Lowers blood cholesterol
- Inhibits triglyceride absorption
- Has an antiobesity affect
- Enhances fat metabolism and insulin sensitivity
- Provides excellent defense against heart disease and diabetes
- Reduces allergic conditions by blocking the release of histamine, which controls allergic reactions
- Protects the colon against free-radical damage
- Works as a cancer preventive
- Helps to prevent bone loss in menopausal osteoporosis

Upon returning to the United States after visiting with Professor Yasargil, I experienced the one major side affect of consuming lots of apples. Attempting to replicate his consumption of 1 to 1.5 pounds per day, I developed GI problems that led me to modify my consumption, beginning more slowly and working up to one to three apples per day, which I then tolerated. If you go this route, look for apples that are organic, or at least free of pesticides, and eat them before meals or as a complex carbohydrate snack in the afternoon instead of a candy bar or high-fructose, high-caffeine soda.

2. Concentrated Polyphenols: Xeno Grape Extracts

The Australian Extract

In chapters 7 and 8, I described how Peter Voigt turned the trash of discarded grape skins into treasure by using his extraction technique to make a superconcentrated polyphenol product, which he referred to as the Australian extract. After confirming the extremely high content of polyphenols, including resveratrol, he needed to know if it activated the sirtuins and increased longevity the way resveratrol had done in the Harvard studies conducted by Joseph Baur and David Sinclair. He contacted Baur and requested a yeast life-span analysis. The Australian extract was evaluated and compared with a control product and resveratrol. It was fed to yeast to determine if it could prolong the life span of yeast as much as resveratrol alone. Indeed it did!

Next Voigt contacted an independent lab used by the United States Department of Agriculture and asked it to compare the antioxidant capacity of various juices and a wine marketed for their high antioxidant levels to the Australian extract. The lab used the ORAC (oxygen radical absorbance capacity) analysis, which is the standard for measuring the capacity of antioxidants against the free radicals found in the body. It demonstrated that the superxeno Australian extract with added resveratrol in a red wine grape juice had an antioxidant capacity many times greater than that of other commercially marketed antioxidant juices (Noni juice and XanGo juice) and Cabernet Sauvignon wine.

In a trial of the Australian extract plus resveratrol in sedentary adults, those who took the extract exhibited improved endurance, memory, and reaction time. Peter Voigt is still working on developing a commercially available product.

Powergrape

Discoveries by scientists like Sinclair and Baur about the health benefits from plant sources, especially polyphenols, have not escaped the notice of the nutrition industry. Just as Peter Voigt was drawn to the excitement of grape extracts and their potential health benefits, so were some of the largest manufacturers of health supplements in the world. One of the earliest was the Berkem Group, headquartered in Gardonne, France, with offices and manufacturing facilities in China, Thailand, and the United States. Since its inception in 1964, Berkem has focused on producing polyphenols and, starting in the early 1990s, has been refining the processes of plant nutrient extraction on an industrial scale. The company currently makes plant-based ingredients for the pharmaceutical, nutraceutical, cosmetic, and food industries.

As a French company, Berkem was quite aware of the health benefits of red wine and also the burgeoning scientific reports showing that it was the polyphenols in the red wine—and, therefore, the red grape—that were mostly responsible for these benefits. Unlike Voigt, who had worked with Pinot grapes in southern Australia, the scientists at Berkem decided to use Bordeaux grapes, which surrounded their main office.

Berkem applied a unique hydroalcoholic extraction process to the grapes, using both pure water and food-grade alcohol along with variations in pressure and temperature to obtain specific ratios of the different polyphenols, including resveratrol. The liquid produced was then spray-dried and called Powergrape. The Berkem scientists believed this concentrated polyphenol product would have a powerful antioxidative effect and help to counter the negative effects of stress, smoking, pollution, poor diet, and especially overexertion. Specifically, they believed that during athletic activity, a powerful natural antioxidant might improve or reduce recovery time, reduce the effects of elevated free radicals that occur after extreme exercise, and also enhance endurance.

Powergrape Sports Study

Next they tested their product under conditions that would maximally stress an athlete and then measured blood markers for oxidative stress recovery. Berkem scientists used Powergrape, which was formed into both a capsule and a powder, and performed a placebo-controlled clinical study of twenty professional athletes between the ages of eighteen and thirty-four. Over a two-month time frame, 400 milligrams of Powergrape per day were given to one group of athletes, and a similar-looking "dummy" capsule was given to the control group. Both groups continued to perform their sport activity (soccer) and also were asked to undergo specific aerobic exercise endurance tests.

The researchers found a powerful antioxidant effect in the treated group, with a 60 percent increase in vitamin C levels and a 96 percent increase in ubiquinone, a powerful antioxidant involved in energy production in cells. There was also a marked increase in the plasma ORAC value of those athletes taking Powergrape, further indicating its antioxidant potential. Most significantly, the researchers noted a 21 percent increase in physical performance among those taking the Powergrape supplements, compared with the control group. Scientists from the French Agronomic Research Institute (INRA) and Advantage Nutrition indicated that this product could reduce the risk of muscular damage, improve the explosive sports performance during effort, and improve recovery capability, particularly in athletes.

These results were presented at international conferences in 2006 and 2007. On the basis of the positive results, on January 8, 2008, the France-based Naturex corporation acquired Powergrape from Berkem for $9.5 million. Naturex, one of the largest suppliers of plant-based nutraceuticals in the world, plans to market this product for both its energy and its antiaging potential. Powergrape is packed full of powerful xeno factors that appear to have profoundly positive effects on human health, exercise endurance, and exercise recovery.

3. Commercially Available Resveratrol Supplements

At present the resveratrol supplement industry is made up of diverse products from a variety of manufacturers and producers distributed through multiple channels. Go online, and you may quickly become confused by hundreds of different claims and counterclaims; assertions with little documentation about purity, manufacturing processes, sources, and health benefits are rampant. The fact is, very little can be found out from manufacturers or distributors about these claims in order to objectively confirm or repudiate them. Unless we can obtain this information from well-designed human research studies or prove sirtuin activation using laboratory studies, it truly is caveat emptor, or buyer beware, at this stage in the resveratrol story.

That having been said, if you decide to take a resveratrol-containing dietary supplement, the optimal product would have the following characteristics:

- Produced in an oxygen-free environment
- Sealed in airtight bottles and vials

- Stored away from heat
- Made with trans-resveratrol, not cis-resveratrol
- Shown to activate sirtuin activity through professional testing
- Produced by manufacturers who comply with Good Manufacturing Practices (GMP)
- Free from fillers or additives such as sugar, starch, gluten, and artificial colors or flavors

Health Claims—Getting Past the Hype!

"Antiaging, Now in a Pill"

"The Fountain of Youth Has Now Arrived"

"Explains the French Paradox"

These are but a few of the many marketing claims being made by manufacturers of supplements containing resveratrol. Of course, more is better, and the advertising hyperbole continues to rise. Additionally, many companies claim that their products will bring about the same result as the French paradox.

Certainly if lab animals were in the market for a health-improving polyphenol dietary supplement, we could factually say that these supplements:

- Increase longevity
- Increase mitochondria and exercise endurance
- Help you resist weight gain
- Improve insulin sensitivity
- Impede cancer cell growth
- Protect the heart

Also, if human cell lines were purchasing supplements containing resveratrol, they would be glad to hear that these products can:

- Inhibit many human cancer cell lines
- Improve cardiac muscle cells
- Improve insulin sensitivity

For humans the research is still scarce. Besides the James Smoliga study on endurance and the David Boocock study showing that up to a 5-gram dose of purified resveratrol is safe in humans, most human studies have just received funding or are in the early stages of collecting data. The next several years should see an explosion of human polyphenol and resveratrol supplement studies, which hopefully will mirror successful studies in animals.

So what can be said about resveratrol dietary supplements available today? The Food and Drug Administration, which regulates claims by supplement manufacturers or distributors, allows statements that resveratrol and most of the other phytonutrients in plants can act as powerful antioxidants. This is very good news because humans have lost the ability to produce their own antioxidants, such as vitamins C and E, and therefore can obtain them only from the foods we eat. Resveratrol, as an antioxidant, can claim to participate in physiological, biochemical, or cellular processes that inactivate free radicals or prevent free-radical-initiated chemical reactions. This definition, directly from the FDA, has been proved and cited in the many studies presented in this book describing the antioxidant actions of resveratrol and the other polyphenols studied in both animals and humans. The other claim that is important to look for in a resveratrol-containing dietary supplement is whether or not it can activate the sirtuin genes and enzymes as shown in Howitz and Sinclair's 2003 study. If the manufacturer has done the proper testing, this claim can be made.

Because of the hype surrounding resveratrol and the desire of many manufacturers and distributors to strike it rich, rarely do you see the following discussed in the advertisements:

• The source of resveratrol (polygonum, grape skin or seed "blends," or purified sources)
• The concentration and amount of resveratrol
• The dose as based on animal-to-human conversion
• Sirtuin activation

Manufacturing and Testing Resveratrol Dietary Supplements

As we have discussed, there are more then ten thousand different polyphenols found in the plant kingdom. They are generally concentrated in the skins of plants, especially fruit, are often associated with the colored pigment, and often act as plant protection against herbivores, insects, and fungi. Dietary supplements that contain these polyphenols are sensitive to exposure to air, oxidative enzymes, and heat. Just as fruit left on a shelf can spoil, so can resveratrol and other polyphenols spoil during harvesting, manufacturing, and shipping.

Processing and manufacturing resveratrol, one of the most sensitive polyphenols, can lead to significant exposure to oxygen, which causes rapid oxidation and loss of biological function. Testing conducted by Dr. Sinclair led him to state that there are no commercial resveratrol products that are not oxidized; sealed bottles of red wine can provide unoxidized resveratrol, but once opened, they will oxidize rapidly. Some current producers of resveratrol supplements reject this observation and contend that advancements in manufacturing and storage can reduce the oxidation process. Additional methods used by manufacturers to help reduce oxidation include:

- Microscopic phospholipid "wrap" that seals the products in airtight beads
- Sealing supplements in an opaque nitrogen-filled container
- Mixing resveratrol with other polyphenols
- Adding other antioxidants
- Creating a liquid supplement stored in a sealed bottle
- Storing and shipping in refrigerated or frozen container

The two major sources of resveratrol used in supplements are *Polygonum cuspidatum* (Japanese knotweed) fruit skins, such as red grape skins, that are concentrated and made into polyphenol drink and powder blends. The term *blends* is often used in labeling dietary supplements because this allows the manufacturer or distributor to avoid providing the specific amounts of each component in the blend.

Therefore a resveratrol blend may have only the smallest fraction of resveratrol in it.

The production of purified resveratrol extract, generally from *Polygonum cuspidatum,* requires costly manufacturing and refining capabilities. Just as with oil, the amount of refining that goes into the final product will influence the final price. For example, a 50 percent resveratrol product may cost $65 per kilogram, whereas a 98 percent resveratrol product may cost $650 per kilogram. Typically, labels on resveratrol supplements do not cite the purity or the percentage of resveratrol being used. Thus with many dietary supplement products, the consumer is often paying for inert fillers, with low concentrations of resveratrol.

Another compound found in some resveratrol products is emodin. Emodin is a natural resin that historically has been used as an herbal extract for medical treatment. Plants such as rhubarb, aloe and also *polygonum cuspidatum* used to make many commercial resveratrol products generally contain this resin. The resin belongs to a family of compounds called anthraquinones. Natural healers have reported it to have antiviral, immunosuppressive, anti-inflammatory, and anticancer effects. In general, however, it is known to be a natural laxative. Those who take resveratrol supplements that are not highly purified can develop loose stools due to emodin present in the product. Generally this is a short-term problem, but resveratrol that is 98 to 99 percent pure should not contain any significant amount of emodin.

Products containing resveratrol are shipped to various distributors around the world. If proper temperature controls or light- and air-protection containers are not used, these products will oxidize rapidly. Knowledgeable distributors recognize the need for protective packaging and often promote this in their advertising. But whether the same precautions are taken during the actual sourcing and manufacturing is often unknown.

Because of the "buyer beware" reputation often associated with the supplement industry, there are several private watchdog organizations in addition to the FDA and the FCC (Federal Communications Commission) that review product claims. Rarely, however, do they determine whether a product actually contains the amount of resveratrol that it claims to have. ConsumerLab.com, a private company, has attempted to answer this question. ConsumerLab.com performs independent evaluations of consumer vitamins and minerals, and then publishes the results on its website (www.consumerlab.com). As a self-declared certification company, ConsumerLab.com also provides certification (for a fee) for testing a company's product. The product is then placed on its list of Approved Quality products and bears the ConsumerLab.com seal. This means that ConsumerLab.com specifically evaluated the amount of resveratrol listed on the package, the chemical forms of the resveratrol, the presence of any lead or cadmium contamination, and whether the tablet or caplet effectively breaks apart for absorption in the gut.

The results of ConsumerLab.com's analysis of nineteen commercially available products performed in November 2007 revealed three products with significantly less resveratrol than was claimed on the label. There was no significant contamination found in any of the products. Interestingly, the recommended dose ranged from 1 milligram to 1,000 milligrams, and the cost varied from 10 cents to $45 per 100 milligrams of resveratrol.

In general, reports from watchdog organizations and even reviews by the FDA and FCC do not ensure that a resveratrol supplement will mirror the results seen in animal studies. Human studies on several commercially available products—and on some still not available—are currently under way, and will eventually confirm to what degree these products work in people.

There is one research test for resveratrol products that many researchers consider a viable substitute for human testing. It is the capacity of the product to induce sirtuin activation in a lab test. Most dietary supplements containing resveratrol currently claim SIRT1 activation because they contain resveratrol, but to date very few manufacturers have undertaken the expensive testing needed to prove it.

Some resveratrol dietary supplement manufacturers and distributors believe that the Biomol company's testing for sirtuin activation is flawed, and that the best way to determine if nonoxidized trans-resveratrol is present is to perform a photomicrograph (×100) analysis, which can identify trans-resveratrol's specific particle composition. This is like a fingerprint, which can be compared with standard pure trans-resveratrol to determine the amount present. The general industry standard practice, however, has been to use HPLC (high-performance liquid chromatography). HPLC is a laboratory technique used for the separation, identification, purification, and quantification of chemical compounds.

Longevinex is one of the first resveratrol products based on the scientific work of Sinclair, Guarente, and others, and the company has gone to considerable lengths to emphasize the quality of this web-based product. Its capsules are reportedly processed in a nitrogen (nonoxygen) environment, protected from light exposure by placement in an opaque capsule, and then sealed in a foil package. Microencapsulation is used and said to enhance absorption and reduce negative effects from direct exposure to ultraviolet radiation. Also added to the trans-resveratrol are vitamin D_3 and quercetin. The company reports that its tests confirm sirtuin gene activation. The capsules come in 100 milligrams, and one to three per day are recommended, at a cost of approximately $1.23 per capsule.

Biotivia is a resveratrol dietary supplement distributor whose product Bioforte Resveratrol 500 is reported to have 250 milligrams of trans-resveratrol as assessed by HPLC provided by ConsumerLab.com, and by its own photomicrograph (×100) analysis. On the basis of Biotivia's cost of approximately 12 cents per milligram of resveratrol, it appears to have the most inexpensive pricing at this time. Its products are now manufactured in a nitrogen environment and protected from light in a GMP facility. Biotivia maintains that its product has superior bioavailability and promotes NAD and the SIRT1–4 longevity enzymes. (NAD increases sirtuin activity and the SIRT1–4 longevity enzymes.)

There is hope that the industry has begun to understand the unique manufacturing, storage, and testing issues associated with resveratrol. In January 2008 RevGenetics, an importer of self-reported 99 percent pure resveratrol, announced its results for sirtuin activation as tested by the Biomol laboratory. The company states that its product, X1000, activated sirtuins at a level comparable to the pharmaceutical-grade resveratrol used by Biomol. In addition, RevGenetics reports that it performs independent testing on each shipment of resveratrol it imports and that its manufacturing facilities are GMP compliant, indicating high-quality manufacturing and processing. This all comes at a price. X1000, which is 990 milligrams of trans-resveratrol, is currently priced at $95 for thirty capsules (a thirty-day supply). Still, the cost per milligram ranks it as one of the least expensive resveratrol products on the market. Whether a daily human dose of 990 milligrams is the correct amount is still controversial, but RevGenetics does offer a variety of doses, starting at 300 milligrams per capsule of 99 percent pure resveratrol.

TABLE 9. Partial List of Available Resveratrol Dietary Supplements

Distributor	Product Name	Amount of Resveratrol
Arkopharma	French Paradox	1 mg
Biotivia	Resveratrol Bioforte	250 mg
Country Life	Resveratrol Plus Antioxidant	100 mg
Douglas Laboratories	Resvera-Gold	2.5 mg
Duplin Vineyards	NutraGrape	0.01 mg
Invite Health	Resveratrol HX	100 mg
Jarrow Formulas	Resveratrol-100	100 mg
Life Extension	Resveratrol	100 mg, 250 mg
New Chapter	Zyflamend	6.4 mg
Paradise Herbs	Resveratrol	15 mg
Pure Encapsulations	Resveratrol	40 mg
Renaissance Health Publishing	Revatrol	100 mg
Resveratrol Partners	Longevinex	100 mg
RevGenetics	X1000	990 mg
Solaray	Resveratrol	15 mg
Source Naturals	Resveratrol	20 mg

(continued)

Distributor	Product Name	Amount of Resveratrol
Swanson Health Products	High Potency Resveratrol	50 mg
Vitamin Research Products	Resveratrol	300 mg
Shaklee Corporation	Vivix	100 mg

Note: If both trans-resveratrol and total resveratrol are listed, the trans amount will be shown. All resveratrol amounts are self-reported by the distributor. The amount of resveratrol listed is based on the label's daily serving size.

This table is a limited representation of perhaps two hundred or more resveratrol-containing dietary supplements in both liquid and capsule form. It is only a snapshot in time of distributors and products that come and go almost daily in this market. In addition to this limited list, almost every major vitamin and supplement wholesaler and retailer possesses its own brand name of resveratrol-containing supplements.

This list does not represent an endorsement of any product listed. It should be noted that the resveratrol (greater than 98 percent pure) purchased and used by Baur and Sinclair in their research on obese mice was from Orchid Pharmaceuticals of Aurangabad, India. There is no indication in any of the consumer materials of any current dietary supplement manufacturer or distributor that this is also the source of its resveratrol.

See table 9 for a partial list of dietary supplements containing resveratrol.

Many companies have taken Dr. Sinclair's critical remarks about the inactivity of various supplements as a challenge and are addressing areas of resveratrol purity, oxidation risk, and retained biological function. As we've seen, several cutting-edge companies like Longevinex, Biotivia, RevGenetics, and others are attempting to prove that their dietary supplements contain biologically active resveratrol. The current standard should at least include quantified amounts of trans-resveratrol content using HPLC and lab certification of sirtuin activity. Recently Longevinex has used a gene chip about the size of a credit card, which provides data on the expression level of more than twenty thousand genes, in order to demonstrate that this product has powerful gene activating capabilities. Several resveratrol-containing dietary supplements are now being used in human trials, which will provide the definitive answer regarding effectiveness in people. Biotivia, for example, is using its product in cancer research studies in India.

Mixed Polyphenol Product

Vivix™

There is growing scientific evidence that a combination of resveratrol and other potent polyphenols might provide improved health benefits due to the synergistic properties of different polyphenols from different plant sources. Shaklee Corporation, a direct selling nutrition company has recently released a product called Vivix™, which is described as a cellular anti-aging tonic. It contains a multi-source polyphenol blend. In conversations with the company, they state that the blend includes 100 mg of 98 percent pure resveratrol from *Polygonum cuspidatum* along with a proprietary extract derived from the fresh pomace of muscadine grapes (*Vitis rotundifolia*). The company recommends 5 ml per day of Vivix, which they state is equivalent to the amount of resveratrol found in 100 glasses of pinot noir red wine. The muscadine polyphenols in this blended product along with the added resveratrol, European elderberry extract, and purple carrot extract will increase the total overall polyphenol content of this product. A month's supply will cost a member $85.

In Shaklee's accompanying literature for Vivix they state that the Vivix ingredients were shown in a laboratory study to be 10 times more powerful in slowing a key mechanism of cellular aging than resveratrol alone. No specific studies are listed but here they appear to be recognizing that resveratrol may work better in people as a mixture of complementary polyphenols. They also have focused on leveraging the benefits of the muscadine grape in their product.

4. Pharmaceutical-Grade Resveratrol—Calorie Restriction, Genes, and Drugs

Earlier I explained how the stress of calorie restriction activates the sirtuin gene in order to increase our chances of survival. This stress activates another set of genes, leading to the formation of a potent hormone called *ghrelin,* which has powerful effects on appetite and plays a major role in regulating blood sugar, fat, and body composition. The discoveries of sirtuin genes' role in health and longevity, and ghrelin's regulation of appetite, have prompted entrepreneurial efforts to capitalize on these findings by some of the stars of antiaging research.

In 1999 Drs. Cynthia Kenyon and Lenny Guarente founded a company they named Elixir Pharmaceuticals. They knew that dieters display elevated ghrelin levels and have a greater appetite and hunger than they did before dieting, which may explain why dieters who lose weight often gain it back. Kenyon and Guarente theorized that if they could develop drugs to decrease or block ghrelin levels, they might have discovered the ultimate appetite suppressant and weight-loss solution. Conversely, if they could devise drugs that would mimic ghrelin's action, they might be able to stimulate appetite in people wasting away from aging, cancer, heart failure, or eating disorders, as well as prevent and manage diabetes. In its initial public offering to raise $86 million, Elixir asserted that its researchers "mine the pathways involved in the regulation of aging discovered by our founders."

Influenced by Kenyon and Guarente, David Sinclair also contracted entrepreneurial fever. In 2003 he was approached by venture capitalist Christoph Westphal, known for "conjuring up dreams that spellbind investors," as *Fortune* magazine put it. Together they cofounded a biotech start-up, Sirtris Pharmaceuticals, in 2004. The company's mission is to discover and develop small-molecule drugs that, like resveratrol, treat the diseases of aging based on sirtuin gene activation. With this goal, they quickly raised an initial $103 million in funding from private venture investors, and in May 2007 they raised another $60 million in their initial public offering.

Both companies, Elixir and Sirtris, have focused on developing compounds to treat type 2 diabetes. This type represents 90 percent of all diagnosed diabetic patients, and in the United States it is approximately a $10 billion business. Sirtris intends to develop a proprietary formulation of resveratrol to increase insulin sensitivity, reduce blood sugar, and maintain stable body weight. Elixir has taken a different approach. It hopes to improve insulin sensitivity, blood sugar, body weight, and other factors associated with diabetes by manipulating the genes that control appetite. In the meantime, Elixir has licensed a diabetes drug that has nothing to do with sirtuins but has already been approved in Japan; the company is trying to get this drug approved in the United States while simultaneously pursing research on ghrelin.

At the present time in the Elixir-Sirtris rivalry, Sirtris appears to be leading when it comes to developing drugs that mimic the beneficial effects of calorie restriction and resveratrol. Indeed, in November 2007, after a one-year hiatus from Elixir, Lenny Guarente joined Sirtris as cochairman of its scientific advisory board.

In a short time, the scientific achievements of Sirtris have been outstanding. In November 2007 Sirtris and its equity partner Harvard announced in the journal *Nature* the results of testing their proprietary resveratrol compound. They demonstrated in diabetic rodent models that their compound could decrease insulin resistance and improve sugar metabolism and insulin sensitivity—comparable to the findings previously reported with natural resveratrol in a similarly designed animal study.

In 2006 Sirtris initiated a clinical study with type 2 diabetics. In January 2008 the company announced not only that its first product, SRT-501, was found to be safe and well tolerated in humans, but that it had significantly lowered blood sugar and increased insulin sensitivity in a twenty-eight-day clinical trial. In the study, oral doses of either 2,500 milligrams or 5,000 milligrams of its resveratrol-like compound were given once daily to patients with type 2 diabetes. There were no serious side effects or complications related to these very high doses. Peter Elliott, the senior vice president of development of Sirtris, stated, "This is the first time that a small molecule targeting sirtuins, the genes which control the aging process, has shown efficacy in the disease of aging."

Anticipating uses beyond diabetes for its resveratrol-like product, Sirtris Pharmaceuticals recently announced a collaboration with the National Cancer Institute (NCI). Scientists from both institutions will immediately begin testing the anticancer impact of the SRT-501 compound in well-established cancer cell lines at the NIH. The cell lines to be tested include some of the most common cancer types, such as colorectal, liver, breast, and lung. Additionally, mouse tumor models will be used to determine if the compound reduces or limits the growth of tumor cells in these well-established rodent models.

Molecular biologists at Sirtris have tested five hundred thousand molecules in their search for some that would have the same effect as resveratrol on the sirtuin gene. Their hope is that the discovery of resveratrol mimetics will have implications well beyond diabetes. As Sinclair said, "We will make a drug to treat one disease, but it will, as an added bonus, protect you against most of the other diseases of the Western world." Sirtris is now conducting human studies comparing the effectiveness of SRT-501 with that of the drug metformin, the current first-line treatment for type 2 diabetes.

On April 22, 2008, the labors and risk taking of David Sinclair, Christoph Westphal, and other Sirtris investors were vindicated when GlaxoSmithKline, a giant in the pharmaceutical industry, purchased Sirtris for $720 million. Dr. Moncef Slaoui, chairman of research and development for GlaxoSmithKline, called the modulation of SIRT enzymes as demonstrated by Sinclair "a transformational science" that could address diseases such as diabetes, muscle wasting, and neurodegenerative disease of the brain.

The Pharmaceutical Problems

Just as I have pointed out the problems associated with the natural compounds of resveratrol—source, extraction process, manufacturing, bioavailability, dosing, and cost—there are similar drawbacks to artificially constructed pharmaceutical agents that mimic the effects of resveratrol. Even if we assume the amazing development of a pill that will prevent or treat major diseases and concurrently prolong life, it will still take another five to seven years to move it through the FDA approval process—not to mention the price tag of an additional $700 million to $1 billion. Assuming all goes well, the cost of a doctor-written prescription would have to be high, but then, who wouldn't sell the farm to get it if it truly worked!

The commitment of those pursuing this pharmaceutical solution is unquestioned. Certainly a specific drug with known safety, bioavailability, and dosage schedules would be desirable. If approved by the FDA, pharmaceuticals can be marketed and advertised to treat specific diseases unlike nutraceuticals that can be labeled only "to promote health."

It is also true, however, that virtually all of the studies using natural resveratrol and other plant-derived polyphenols have already demonstrated therapeutic benefits against the same diseases targeted by pharmaceutical companies. They have also increased longevity in all of the animals studied. Although many human studies are under way, they have not yet confirmed these animal observations. But there is increased confidence that the agents will have the same biological effects on people as they do on animals. There is also confidence that these natural products are safe even when taken in large, concentrated dosages.

The question to be addressed is: would plant products (botanicals), when prepared under similar standards as drugs, compete with drug development by pharmaceutical companies? Based on the thousands of studies I have reviewed, my personal belief is that there are opportunities for the supplement products discussed earlier in this chapter to attain at least some of the benefits sought by pharmaceutical companies.

Indeed, GlaxoSmithKline has the option of putting its proprietary resveratrol formulation SRT-501 on the market immediately as a nutraceutical, thereby bypassing the need for FDA approval. However, then it could not make any treatment claims for specific diseases. Dr. Patrick Vallance, head of drug discovery for GSK, stated, "We haven't made any decisions, but that clearly is an option."

There are many competing forces in the rapidly flowing resveratrol river. The pharmaceutical industry, regulated by the Food and Drug Administration (FDA), is not interested in (and may even be opposed to) a natural product that potentially has druglike actions. Nutraceutical manufacturers, on the other hand, are exempt from the FDA drug approval process under the Dietary Supplement Health and Education Act (DSHEA), and are not required to go through pre-market approval.

However, the FDA has enforcement authority over the dietary supplement industry and precludes manufacturers and distributors from making unapproved claims for the treatment or cure of medical conditions and diseases. Furthermore, DSHEA provided FDA with additional enforcement authority, including the ability to remove from the market products the agency deems unsafe or an unreasonable risk. Under the regulations, manufacturers are required to have adequate scientific substantiation for their marketing claims. Having seen both a pharmaceutical manufacturing plant as a board member of Mylan Laboratories, one of the largest generic drug manufactures in the world, and a dietary supplement facility used by General Nutrition Corporation, with whom I participate as a medical advisor, I am assured that the manufacturing standards are virtually identical.

As with any industry, there are some unscrupulous companies that make exaggerated claims. However, these false and misleading claims are prohibited by extensive regulations and enforced by the FDA and FTC.

In the meantime, what is a person to do? Drink wine, eat dark chocolate, sip tea, eat an apple a day, take a concentrated grape skin product or a resveratrol supplement from a reputable company, and pursue balance in one's diet and life—as we will discuss in chapters 19 and 20.

Chapter 19

The Four-Step Xeno Longevity/ Weight-Loss Program

*The great error of our day in the treatment of humans is that
some physicians separate treatment of psyche from treatment
of body.*

—PLATO, 428–347 BC

After reading the title of this chapter, you may be thinking, "What, another diet, after you've already listed a hundred that don't work?" When I began this book, I had no intention of putting together a diet plan, having been through so many of them unsuccessfully myself; for me the point has been seeing diet as just one of a number of keys to a balanced life. Also, I could not ignore a consistent finding in my research: obesity and inflammation are major factors underlying almost all diseases, from cancer to depression. Without successfully addressing these factors, it is unlikely that any pill or nutrient will contribute significantly to a healthier and longer life—the goal of this book.

Several additional factors prompted me to formulate a weight-loss program—not just a diet—that I have personally found successful. These include the following:

1. Inflammation, stress, addiction, and emotional and hormonal disorders are major contributors to weight gain.

2. Xeno factors such as resveratrol, quercetin, and other polyphenols enable animals to maintain a normal weight with increased energy despite eating a high-fat, high-calorie diet.

3. These same molecules have potent anti-inflammatory, anticancer, and antiaging benefits.

4. A balanced life is every bit as important as a balanced diet.

With these observations in hand, it seemed a natural progression to apply what we know about diseases, weight loss, and xeno factors in a practical, useful way.

The difference between the Xeno Program and other diets is that the Xeno Program requires a commitment not only to balance your diet but to balance your life. Health and longevity require both. Having experienced some major periods of imbalance in my own life, I believe this program is optimal because it considers all the various causes of weight gain—hormonal, genetic, inflammatory, and psychological—and provides a solution for each. There are four parts to the program:

1. A baseline evaluation
2. A reasonable exercise program
3. Eating an anti-inflammatory, organic (when possible) diet
4. Supplementation with xeno factors and resveratrol

With this program, weight loss and health occur as secondary events, while we pursue more pleasant things than dieting!

Step 1: Baseline Evaluation

Before moving on to my balancing program, you will need a baseline medical evaluation by a doctor, particularly if you are over forty-five or if you have preexisting health problems. Factors that may be contributing to weight gain should be identified. Also, assessment of the amount of damage already done to the body should be measured so that improvement can subsequently be documented.

Assessment of hormonal levels by way of a simple blood test is essential because abnormal levels may contribute to weight gain and may need to be corrected up front. Thyroid dysfunction is one of the most frequent problems discovered in overweight patients. The thyroid gland, a butterfly-shaped clump of tissue just under the voice box in the throat, produces an active hormone that has profound effects on the body. The symptoms of thyroid deficiency include fatigue, increased weight gain, hair loss, dry skin and nails, and many others. If thyroid hormone is deficient, taking an oral replacement can lead to dramatic weight loss with little dietary intervention.

The hemoglobin A1C (HgA1C) blood test is one of the best tests to determine the cumulative effects of high levels of blood sugar. It measures the amount of glucose binding to the hemoglobin of red blood cells. A longer and higher exposure to glucose in the blood will lead to a higher reading. Blood sugar, HgA1C levels, and insulin levels are measured to predict the propensity for type 2 diabetes—if it has not already developed. If one is under chronic, intense stress, a test measuring cortisol also may shed light on the cause as well as the consequences of excessive weight. Other hormone levels to be considered include growth hormone, estrogen, and testosterone.

A lipid profile that includes total cholesterol, LDL cholesterol, HDL cholesterol, triglycerides, and the subfractions of cholesterol will provide useful baseline values. Measurement of the waist-to-hip ratio is a low-tech test that is predictive of insulin resistance. You or your doctor simply divides the waist measurement at the belly button level by the hip measurement at the widest point over the hips. For women this number should be 0.8 or less; for men, less than 0.9; values above this are frequently associated with insulin resistance and type 2 diabetes.

As previously discussed, excessive fat leads to inflammation in the body. There are now several measurable substances that indicate the amount of inflammation; markers that can be seen to improve with weight loss and exercise. These inflammatory markers include the high-sensitivity C-reactive protein, also called "cardio CRP." Measurements of homocystine and fibrinogen are markers of cardiovascular risk. Other sophisticated but less frequently used blood tests assess various cytokines, which are proteins that participate in the inflamma-tory process in our heart, brain, and joints.

Before embarking on an exercise program, those of us over the age of forty-five, especially if sedentary, should undergo a stress test. This is easily performed in a doctor's office by walking on a treadmill to assess heart rate, heart rhythm, and blood pressure during the exer-cise. This is an important baseline measurement procedure to detect hidden coronary artery disease prior to major exertion.

I routinely recommend measurement of arachidonic acid (AA), a powerful inflammatory agent, as well as the amount of essential fatty acids in the blood. The ratio of this potentially harmful substance (AA) to the healthy essential fatty acids (such as EPA and DHA—omega-3 fatty acids—from fish and fish oil) is one of the best indicators of car-diovascular risk. The higher the arachidonic acid level compared with omega-3 essential fatty acids, the greater the risk. An estimated 40 per-cent of Americans are deficient in omega-3s. This deficiency is easily corrected with fish oil supplements.

Optional tests, depending on each patient, include specific tests for allergies to gluten and other foods; tests for infections such as *Heli-cobacter pylori,* which is the cause of ulcers; and measurements of minerals and vitamins to assess specific deficiencies.

All of these tests are best taken in conjunction with a physician after a comprehensive history and physical examination. This allows us to pinpoint areas of possible trouble and obtain the appropriate tests for diagnostic and baseline evaluation.

The Most Important Lab Tests
Physical Exam

Vital signs: blood pressure, heart rate, and temperature

Baseline weight

Body mass index (BMI)*

Percentage of body fat

*[BMI—weight kg (e.g., 68) ÷ height meters (e.g., 165 cm or 1.65 m) = 24.98 BMI; or google BMI calculation on the internet. Over 30 = overweight.]

Baseline Lab Tests

Blood count, to assess for anemia/infection

Chemistry screen, to assess liver and kidney function

Cholesterol testing, to assess lipid levels

Endocrine Tests

Thyroid function

Fasting blood sugar level

Cortisol levels

Inflammatory Markers

C-reactive protein

Other Tests

(May be recommended by your health-care provider)

Stress test

Chest X-ray

Prostatic-specific antigen (PSA), for men

Step 2: How to Attain a Balanced Life— The Mind-Body Connection

Later in this chapter, I will discuss the "easy" part of my weight-loss plan: the use of diet, xeno factors, and supplements. But something is surely wrong, and the problem is more difficult than "taking a pill for every ill," when 90 percent to 95 percent of people who diet regain the weight—or add even more—only a few years after starting any of the hundreds of available diet plans. The problem, from my perspective, is much more closely connected to the fact that our lives are out of balance than to the idea that our diets are low-fat, high-fat, low-carb, high-carb, high-grapefruit, or even high-sex, as often proposed.

We now have scientific confirmation that food is addictive. My belief is that in many cases, we succumb to this addiction due to the frustrations, fears, anxiety, depression, and anger that result from im-

balance or dissatisfaction in our lives. Seeking relief from these negative feelings (seeking more of the neurotransmitters dopamine and
serotonin), we turn to feel-good foods high in carbs and fat. Yet mental
health experts have confirmed that these distressing emotional states
are temporarily but never fully satisfied by eating—a condition much
like that of the brain-damaged patient with Klüver-Bucy syndrome
whom I told you about in chapter 17.

If diets fail because we are addicted to food, and if food addiction
is secondary to the unbalanced lives that are epidemic in our society,
how do we go about righting the imbalance? I have pondered this
question long and often in the course of my own intermittently unbalanced life, and I have come up with a formula that I have shared with
my patients as well as thousands of patients and physicians. This formula, if followed, will lead to a balanced life—and, secondarily, to
weight loss. It has been used successfully by tens of thousands of
people. The formula was first passed on to me by William Danforth,
founder and chairman of the Ralston Purina Company, in his book
I Dare You! In it he challenges the reader to lead a four-square life; and
if one does, the guaranteed result is a life in balance.

I received the book at my high school graduation. Although I read
it at the time, I didn't fully appreciate its significance until twenty years
later. Up until then, I had spent my life striving to get more done and to
do it faster and better than anyone else—at times by neglecting my
family, my health, and my God. Then in the same week, I lost my father
to a heart attack and my wife and family to divorce, and I became so
depressed that I temporarily gave up my job as a university professor
of neurosurgery. I happened to pick up Danforth's book while clean-
ing my bookshelves, I reread it, and I have followed his prescription to
this day.

His instructions called for drawing a square and labeling the sides
with the four major components of our life: work, family/social, spiritual, and physical (see figure 18).

Next I had to redraw the square with the length of each side pro-
portional to how much time and effort I actually put into each aspect
of my life. At that time, mine looked like figure 19.

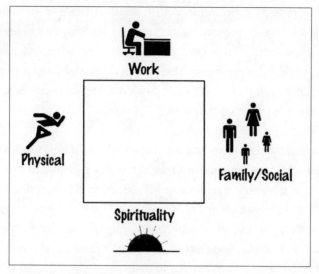

FIGURE 18 William Danforth's balanced life: all sides equal.

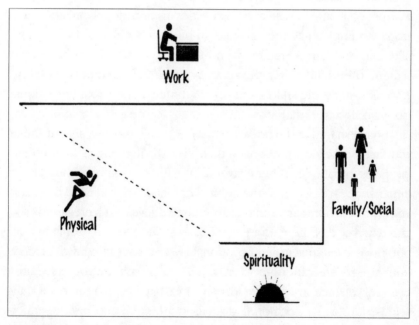

FIGURE 19 Life out of balance: too much work, little to no family/social and spirituality, no physical.

This simple graphic depiction of the imbalance in my life had a huge impact on me. Looking at my own square that first time, I could see that my twenty-five-pound weight gain, my depression, and my emotional distress were due to the lopsided imbalance in my spiritual, physical, and family/social lives. My work had become my escape from facing what was going on in my life.

In this desperate time, I received a phone call from an old friend who asked me to join him for a run. Although I had never enjoyed running, we talked and jogged four laps around a high school football field. To my amazement, not only had I jogged a whole mile—something I had not done since college—but at the end of that day, I also, for the first time in months, slept through the night. The next day, I repeated the run alone, and over subsequent weeks I extended it to the point where the local townspeople must have thought I was Forrest Gump! Eventually I ran my first 10-kilometer race. While I was training, my mood improved, my weight started to melt away (without dieting), my brain regained its old level of function, and I was able to return to neurosurgery after a year of trying to save my father's dilapidated truck stop by pumping gas and making hamburgers. I added swimming and biking to my exercise regimen, and I have now completed more than sixty triathlons, including the Hawaiian Ironman event in Kona (swim 2.4 miles, cycle 112 miles, and run 26.2 miles) and four international Ironman distance triathlons.

I have shared this story with many people, who also shared theirs with me. Some have rebalanced their lives through more involvement on the spiritual side. Others have made efforts to improve their family dimension. Work is often the culprit that leads to truncated time and energy in the other areas of our lives. Over the years, I have discovered that when one of these four is "off," I can still function reasonably well, but if two are deficient, my emotional life becomes filled with anxiety, depression, frustration, or even anger—at myself and others. And I overeat! Balance in our lives doesn't just happen. It requires a conscious (left brain) decision and focused attention and insight, which are often absent. The visual aid of the square brings them into focus.

The great news is that science has discovered that our thoughts actually change the structure of our brain. Dr. Jeffrey Schwartz, a neuroscientist at the University of California, Los Angeles, and author of *The Mind and the Brain,* used PET (positron-emission tomography) scans to study the brains of patients severely affected with obsessive-compulsive disorders. He showed that focused attention not only markedly improved the behavior of his OCD patients but actually changed their brain circuitry and structure. This is a radical new concept because until recently, what was encoded or imprinted in the brain was considered immutable. I believe this transformative focus directed to altering the sides of our square can permanently change our brain anatomy and function.

This concept of attaining balance is as old as humanity itself. All natural systems, from rain forests to killifish, struggle to maintain equilibrium in the face of external and internal forces. Our genes and our brains have been programmed over hundreds of thousands of years to seek balance, and thereby happiness. The same anxiety, fear, and apprehension that we feel, mediated in the frontal/temporal lobes, were also experienced by our ancestors, whose brains were wired just like ours. The difference is that today, with virtually unlimited food resources at our disposal, a marked decrease in exercise, and the tremendous stresses of work and family, we are experiencing an epidemic of obesity unlike anything in human history. Under stress, we reach for comfort foods high in fat and sugar, and the addiction is reinforced.

Food addiction will never be cured by a specific diet, as scientific studies have now clearly established. Reprogramming our brains to prevent or escape addiction will occur only as a side effect of: (1) increased physical activity, which actually modifies and creates new brain connections; (2) a focus on developing our spiritual life, which reduces the destructive stress hormones; (3) strengthening our family and social relationships; and (4) being judicious about how much time and energy go into our work. This discussion of success in dieting and its implications for longevity reminds me of the Austrian psychologist Viktor Frankl, who wrote in his book *Man's Search for Meaning* about how we find happiness: Frankl said, "Don't aim at success [e.g., in dieting]—the more you aim at it and make it a target, the more you're going to miss it. For success [e.g., in dieting], like happiness, cannot be pursued; it must ensue . . . as the unintended side effect of one's personal dedication to a course greater than one's self." I believe that the course to which we must dedicate ourselves is the pursuit of a balanced life. Weight loss, health, and longevity will then ensue as an "unintended side effect"!

Getting Balance in Your Life

Work

In Chinese medicine, it is said that human beings are like batteries: we have a finite amount of energy, and when that energy is used up, we die. In Japan, *karoshi* means "death by overwork." Karoshi's victims, and there are ten thousand each year, work over one hundred hours a week, every week and every month, much as I did, and then die precipitately of heart attacks or strokes secondary to stress. Stress has replaced infectious agents of disease as the primary menace to health in Japan, and in all of Western society.

Nobody ever talks about the American *leisure* ethic. America is a work-oriented culture. We value being successful, being ambitious, and being well off financially, and we work to be those things. In fact, society encourages imbalance as the way to "success." Mihaly Csikszentmihalyi, a professor and former chairman of the department of psychology at the University of Chicago, summed it up this way: "Society applauds imbalance, honoring us for self-sacrifice and awarding financial success. But these achievements are won at times at the cost of diminution of 'self' and personality. We are more useful to society when a small part of us is overdeveloped than when we are whole people." That may be well and good for society, but a workweek of eighty to one hundred hours doesn't make for a whole person—or for a balanced, happy life.

The formula given for success in our culture is:

$$\frac{Accomplishments + accumulations + recognition}{age} = success$$

A healthier view is:

Right relationships + right purposes + balance in our lives = success.

Here are some ways, easier said than done, to keep work from taking over your life:

- Write all nonwork commitments on your work calendar. This includes dates with your spouse, kids' soccer games, and family game night. Don't allow work obligations to supersede these.
- Underpromise and overdeliver. Give yourself more time for each project than you think it will take. Your stress level will go way down.
- Work with your supervisor, coworkers, and company to set reasonable expectations for the workweek of salaried employees. If you work by the hour, don't be seduced by overtime or weekend projects.
- Take all your vacation and comp/personal time each year.
- Take a mental health day at least once per quarter and just goof off.

Family/Social

The time we spend with others includes some of the most valuable hours of our lives. Make the most of it.

- Schedule time weekly with immediate family, and monthly with extended family. Plan game nights, weekend activities that include mild to moderate exercise, and vacations together.
- Cultivate at least one or two intimate friendships outside your family circle. Find people with whom you can laugh and cry.
- Each month, volunteer to help others in some way. This is a great activity to do with friends and family.
- A few times a year, take a class or workshop where you'll meet new people with similar interests.

Spirituality/Meditation

Most people grasp the notion of getting fit through physical training and exercise. Scientists now understand how and why active participation in religious practices and meditation alleviates anxiety and stress, and also can enhance mental skills. The repetition of the rosary, the practice of Buddhist meditation, immersion in the Koran, and balancing *keva* and *kavanah* in Jewish liturgy—all these are forms of "mindfulness" and nonjudgmental "awareness." I believe this is where all religions intersect to focus the mind and to change neural connections in the brain. Indeed, in 2008, scientists at the University of Wisconsin reported that positive emotions like compassion and loving-kindness can be learned, just like playing a musical instrument or a sport. Even more strikingly, brain scans showed that practicing meditation dramatically changed the brain circuits for emotion and feeling. When practiced regularly, religion and spirituality enable us to cultivate a longer attention span, develop emotional stability, and feel more content with what we have rather than focusing on what's missing in our lives.

Spirituality, I have found, is the least recognized deficiency for those on the road to success. Rather than drawing a square, I sometimes draw a triangle (see figure 20) with spirituality in the center, in-

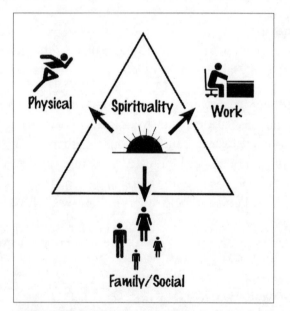

FIGURE 20 This triangle shows the central position of spirituality in our lives.

forming all three other areas of life: work, family/social, and physical. To me this represents the way life works best.

Dr. Jon Kabat-Zinn, founder of the pioneering Stress Reduction Clinic at the University of Massachusetts Medical Center, commented on the insight that comes from meditation: "Awareness gives you your life back, and then you can decide what to do with it."

Here are some suggestions for developing the spiritual component of your life:

- Begin to practice daily prayer or meditation, a time of quiet reflection. Some people choose structured practices, such as following the breath or repeating a mantra or religious phrase. Others just like to sit quietly with a cup of tea and look out the window. Having a time each day—as little as fifteen minutes—when we can let our minds and bodies rest from constant activity does wonders for our mental health.
- Many people find that exploring their creative side puts them in touch with their spiritual nature as well. Consider a hobby that gets you out in nature, like drawing or photography. Try abstract painting or keep a journal as a way to express your feelings and beliefs.
- Develop a practice of gratitude for your many blessings, however large or small they may be.
- Practice directing kindness and compassion toward those who irritate and annoy you. Let people into traffic or the checkout line. Volunteer at a soup kitchen or neighborhood cleanup.
- Be generous with your time and money.
- Experience the spiritual aspects of walking, jogging, swimming, and spontaneous play.
- Focus your attention on the activity at hand and on the present moment. Live in the now.

Physical

As a species, we have never been more sedentary. And most scientists agree that the combination of oversize meals and underused bodies is a major contributor to our obesity epidemic and its many associated ills. An active adult typically burns between 2,000 and 3,000 calories a day through ordinary activity. A Big Mac with fries and a Coke may contain two-thirds of this in one meal! To burn that off would require walking for one and a half hours, swimming one and a half miles, or jogging five miles at an eight-minute-per-mile pace.

Since most weight gain occurs because we eat more calories than we burn, it is obvious that by decreasing how many calories we consume every day, we will reduce or at least maintain our present weight. Indeed, if there is a magic bullet that can cure or prevent many of the diseases we experience, it is exercise. Its benefits are almost innumerable. Here are just a few confirmed by scientific studies.

- Reduces inflammation, and by doing so, improves cardiovascular, joint, brain, and metabolic health.
- Improves the body's ability to detoxify itself, to remove the buildup of waste in the blood and muscles.
- Normalizes hormonal rhythms; increases libido, decreases insulin sensitivity, and increases carbohydrate utilization, among other effects.
- Improves mental balance; elevates mood, reduces depression and anxiety.
- Reduces irritability and increases patience.
- Builds self-confidence and self-esteem.
- Helps the body reach and maintain a healthy weight.
- Supports recovery from food addiction by increasing the release of dopamine.
- For those aged seventy, increases the chance of reaching ninety by nearly half.

If these benefits could be obtained in a pill, everyone would rush to take it!

The remarkable thing is that even a small amount of exercise can be of great benefit.

Four components contribute to physical fitness:

1. Cardiovascular (aerobic) conditioning
2. Strengthening muscles (and, secondarily, bone)

3. Flexibility (stretches)
4. Balance and agility

For cardiovascular fitness, five to ten minutes a day of walking on level ground is a good start, with a goal of moving up to thirty minutes per session, five or six days a week. As fitness increases, sixty minutes a day prevents weight gain, and ninety minutes promotes weight loss. Fitness experts all recommend finding several enjoyable activities. Walking, swimming, jogging, biking, using a treadmill or elliptical machine, rowing, skating, bouncing on a trampoline, and hiking are just a few of the possibilities. Like to dance? Dancing, particularly the tango, is considered one of the best aerobic activities, not only for cardiovascular fitness but also for agility and flexibility.

As we get older, our muscles sag, are replaced by fat, and become soft. Strength training with light weights and stretchy bands, yoga, and Pilates all enhance muscle as well as bone strength. Yoga and Pilates are excellent ways to increase flexibility of joints and muscles; and other simple stretching programs can also go a long way toward increasing flexibility. Try adding five to ten minutes of stretching to the end of a cardio workout. Take a five-minute break from the computer or the television every hour to bend at the waist, do a deep knee bend or two, and stretch your arms up and back. Most of our modern activities are forward in the body (arms, hands in front of the torso). It's important to stretch the other way with your back straightened and your head, arms, and shoulders back.

Agility and balance become even more important as we age. The Chinese practices of qi gong and tai chi are excellent ways to enhance your balance and flexibility. Yoga poses also engage balance, as do any number of exercises involving the large, inexpensive exercise balls that are now available everywhere. What's more, many internet sites provide diagrams or short videos of flexibility, balance, and agility exercises. Adding one balance exercise to your workout routine can work wonders.

Here are some ideas for getting more physical and having fun as you balance your life:

- Exercise with a friend. Find someone who's committed to being more physical and is willing to share accountability with you. Just as obesity is "contagious," so is weight loss. Thin or motivated friends help!
- Schedule your exercise times into your day planner. Then keep those appointments with as much integrity as you would an appointment with your doctor or accountant.
- Walk, walk, walk. Upstairs, downstairs, to the store, around the block, to the movies. Hike in the woods, on the beach. Just get moving.
- Take a class in something physical: dance, karate, qi gong, yoga, kickboxing, tai chi.
- Do something active with your kids, your spouse, or your workmates.

Step 3: The Xeno Diet

"Eat less and work out"—probably the most unwelcome advice an overweight, sedentary person seeking a weight-loss plan can hear. But *what* to eat? Michael Pollan, in his recent best-selling book *In Defense of Food,* puts it succinctly in his eater's manifesto: "Eat food, not much, mostly plants." I have studied hundreds of recommended diets and tried many. All, in some manner, come down to reduced calories and increased activity for their "revolutionary" plan to reshape our bodies, melt away excess fat, control hunger, decrease appetite, and improve our health *for life.* The hook may be high protein, low carbohydrate, daily grapefruit, or improved sex, but the bottom line is always to balance our diet and physical activity—eat less and work out—just as we balance our lives.

Basis of the Xeno Diet

Our understanding of food has been radically changed by the new sciences of cellular and molecular biology. No longer do we eat just to survive in a hostile environment or as a simple matter of filling our bellies. Food is now recognized as a way to affect our genes and how they function. Dr. Raymond L. Rodriguez, director of the Center of Excellence for Nutritional Genomics at the University of California, Davis, puts it this way: "When you consume a food, your genes are like a Christmas tree; red and green lights that flip on and off and flicker back and forth. My Christmas tree lights differ from yours and flicker at a different rate. Over time, depending on your types of genes and how frequently they are turned on and off, you will either be healthy or in a diseased state."

Micronutrients (vitamins, minerals, and plant phytochemical compounds) and macronutrients (proteins, carbohydrates, and fats) all alter gene expression, for better or worse. Too much of the wrong nutrients, and we develop diabetes, hypertension, and heart attacks. Not enough of the right nutrients, and we develop birth defects (from insufficient folic acid), anemia (from iron deficiency) and cancer (from too little vitamin D). Stress, if it doesn't kill a plant—or a person—can make both healthier and stronger. This is the concept of hormesis in action. It is why a potentially lethal fungal infection in grapes activates the antifungal resveratrol gene, improving survival. It is also why calorie restriction and exercise (both stressors with similar survival-gene activation) can lead to weight loss, disease suppression, and increased longevity—as reported by nutrition pioneer Clive McCay in the 1930s.

Our Xeno (hormetic) Diet focuses on stressed plant compounds (polyphenols) and exercise to activate anti-inflammatory, anticancer, and antiaging genes for a healthier and longer life. The bad news is that our bodies and genes are getting their daily dose of poisons from environmental toxins, trans fats, excess sugar and salt, and specific deficiencies in our Western diet. The good news is that it is never too late to change. Eating less, eating better, and exercising lead to healthy gene activation that can actually reverse inflammation, block cancer, and enhance the quality and length of life.

To determine where we are going with our Xeno Diet, let's look at where we came from. For hundreds of thousands of years, our genes have been activated by specific foods. S. Boyd Eaton, MD, an evolutionary nutrition expert from Emory University, described this food-gene interaction as follows: "We are the heirs of inherited characteristics accrued over millions of years; the vast majority of our biochemistry and physiology is tuned to life conditions [and foods] that existed prior to the advent of agriculture some ten thousand years ago. Genetically our bodies and genes are virtually the same as they were at the end of the Paleolithic period some twenty thousand years ago."

Before the cultivation of grains and the domestication of animals, our genes were activated and modified by the food available. This included wild game, foraged fruit, berries, nuts, leaves, roots, flowers, mushrooms, eggs, and honey. This so-called Paleolithic, or hunter-gatherer, diet contrasts starkly with the typical Western diet, with its processed meat from grain-fed animals, drinks and foods high in sugar and fructose, French fries, refined grains, and dairy and meat products contaminated by hormones and pesticides. This also explains why hundreds of millions of people have allergies and intolerance to lactose (from milk) and gluten (from processed grains). Their genes, despite ten thousand years of conditioning, still haven't adapted to these "new" dietary products.

The diets considered healthiest today are those that most closely resemble the ones that have interacted with our genes over hundreds of thousands of years. The Mediterranean and Asian diets are considered the healthiest. They are high in vegetables, fruits, plants, fish, and poultry, and low in refined grains, sugars, dairy products, red meat, and saturated fats. Olive oil and avocado are the main sources of fat in these diets, and they are healthy, monounsaturated good fats. Water, juices, and moderate amounts of alcohol, primarily red wine, are the drinks of choice. Hundreds of scientific studies prove that a diet rich in polyphenol-containing foods, vegetables, and fish, like the Mediterranean diet, decreases obesity-related diseases like diabetes and also the risk of dying from all Western diseases. Polyphenols are the most abundant antioxidants in these diets, and, as we've seen, they are associated with decreased cancer, heart disease, and stroke.

Those who attempt to lose weight by calorie restriction alone fail more than 90 percent of the time. We believe that adding greater quantities of high-quality foods is a better model. A pound of vegetables is just as filling as a pound of cake, but the cake is full of bad calories, and the vegetables are full of nutrients. Simply put, eliminate those foods that signal the inflammatory- and cancer-provoking gene activation, and add those foods that are xenohormetically protective.

Dr. Jeffrey Bland, an internationally respected nutrition expert, searched for a drug or some other magic bullet for weight loss and health. He concluded, "The best molecules for managing chronic disease will not come from the discoveries of pharmaceutical chemists but, rather, from the laboratory of natural selection in our traditional foods that have been associated with the low incidence of obesity, heart disease, and diabetes." Succinct, correct, and never said better.

Given our various lifestyles and energy needs, one diet does not fit all. A construction worker is going to have different needs for carbohydrate, protein, and fat than a sedentary office worker or a young mother. With our Xeno Diet, the essential components for a healthy lifestyle can be modified for different energy needs.

The Xeno Diet Rx

The following are the essentials of our balanced weight-loss Xeno Diet:

- Subscribe to the 80-20 rule. At least 80 percent of each meal (by weight) should be plant based and no more than 20 percent animal based.
- A list of fruits and vegetables high in xeno-polyphenols is provided in table 10 on page 220 for the 80 percent.
- Protein (the lower on the food chain the better): seaweed→algae→ plants→fish→poultry→mammals. A small piece of fish (not farm raised) is much better than a well-marbled steak. Protein is essential, and fermented soy (tofu, miso, tempeh, tamari), soy protein powders, soy milk, chicken, and other poultry are excellent sources.
- Fat is essential. Good (unsaturated) fats, from fish, fish oil, olive oil, and avocados, are necessary for brain, heart, joint, and immune health. Bad (saturated) fats, from beef, lamb, and pork, for example, should be consumed sparingly. My book *Fish Oil: The Natural Anti-Inflammatory*, cowritten with Jeffrey Bost, is an excellent resource on the health benefits of the omega-3 essential fats DHA and EPA.
- Eat complex carbohydrates, which break down slowly, have a low

glycemic index, and release glucose gradually into the bloodstream. They include most fruits and vegetables; whole grains, breads, and pasta; and legumes such as beans and lentils.

- Avoid simple carbohydrates, which break down rapidly during digestion and have a high glycemic index, such as cornflakes, baked potatoes, white rice, white bread, and sugar-filled items such as candy bars, fructose-laced sodas, and energy drinks.
- Consume 40 to 45 grams a day of fiber from whole grains, leafy greens, beans, lentils, oatmeal, raw vegetables, and fruits.
- Enhance your infection resistance and digestion with lacto-fermented foods (probiotics from yogurt, milk with lactobacillus) and supplements.
- Avoid "white stuff": white flour, white bread, white rice, salt, sugar, and cream sauces.
- Drink red wine (no more than two glasses a day for men and one for women), 6 to 8 ounces a day of grape juice, and tea (green or white, two to five cups per day), and eat 70 percent dark chocolate.

How Much and How Often

In their nationally best-selling book *You: The Owner's Manual*, Michael Roizen, MD, and Mehmet C. Oz, MD, present an Owner's Manual Diet. In it they make several good basic suggestions to be followed with any diet plan:

- Eat when hungry, not famished, and make your last meal at least three hours before bedtime.
- Reduce your plate size from eleven or thirteen inches to nine inches.
- Eat nine handfuls of fruits and vegetables and at least 1 ounce of nuts, whole-grain breads, and high-fiber cereals daily.
- Eat fish (preferably not farm raised) such as salmon, sardines, mackerel, tilapia, and flounder at least three times a week.
- Consider taking the following supplements on a daily basis:
    1. A high-potency multivitamin or another supplements to get at least 1,000 to 2,000 IU of vitamin D; 400 micrograms of folate;

1,200 milligrams of calcium; 400 milligrams of magnesium; 1,000 milligrams of vitamin C; 400 milligrams of vitamin E; and the daily value of other minerals and B vitamins.

2. One baby aspirin daily after age forty.

3. Omega-3 fatty acids (fish oil) containing at least 1 to 2 grams of EPA/DHA per day for those over thirty.

4. Coenzyme Q10: 100 milligrams per day in a nanoparticle-sized product for highest absorption, especially if you're taking statin drugs.

5. Turmeric: 500 milligrams per day. An excellent anti-inflammatory and anticancer agent from the curcumin plant.

6. Probiotics: 5–10 billlion colonies per capsule per day containing *L. acidophilus* and bifidobacteria.

Xeno Diet Tools

Boost Your Polyphenol Intake and Track Your Xeno Score

As previously mentioned, polyphenols are key constituents of foods responsible for many health benefits, including reducing disease risk, controlling inflammation, and promoting healthy aging. The first step that you can take to living the xeno way is to focus on incorporating high-polyphenol foods into your daily diet. Table 10 lists polyphenol-rich foods that should appear regularly on your shopping list. By simply ensuring that at least one of these foods is a part of every meal and snack that you eat, you'll start boosting your polyphenol intake and shifting your diet in the right direction. In the list below, a xeno score from a low of 1 to a high of 5 has been assigned to each food; this score is based upon the food's polyphenol content.

Add up your scores for the day. Shoot for a total daily xeno score of 20 or higher. Although the foods on the list rank as the *best* sources of polyphenols, there are other fruits, vegetables, juices, nuts, and seeds, not listed, that may provide small amounts of polyphenols and other healthy nutrients. It is also important to be aware of the calorie content of foods. Later in this section, I will provide you with calorie-conscious menus and recipes to help you maximize your xeno score along with other healthy components of your diet.

TABLE 10.

Food	Serving Size	Calories	Xeno Score
Red wine	1 glass (6 fl oz)	120	5
Eggplant	2 pieces (½ cup)	17	5
Black grape	17	60	5
Cherry	12 fresh	51	5
Blueberry	¾ cup	62	5
Dark chocolate	2 pieces (Hershey's Kiss size)	50	5
Green tea	1 teacup (6 fl oz)	0–10	5
Pomegranate	1	105	5
Cranberry	¾ cup	35	5
Pear	½ large	60	4
Blackberry	¾ cup	46	4
Black currant	¾ cup	30	4
Dark chocolate coffee bean	2	112	4
Plum	2 small	60	4
Rhubarb	2 stalks	22	3
Soybeans, boiled	½ cup	150	3
Strawberry	1¼ cups	60	3
Orange juice (fresh)	½ cup (4 fl oz)	56	3
Orange	1	60	3
Grapefruit juice	½ cup (4 fl oz)	47	3
Grapefruit	½	60	3
Curly kale	1 cup	36	3
Yellow onion	½ cup	33	3
Apple	1 small	70	3

Food	Serving Size	Calories	Xeno Score
Beans (red or black)	½ cup	110	3
Kiwifruit	1	46	3
Flaxseed	2 tbsp	95	3
Chicory	½ cup	8	3
Black tea	1 teacup (6 fl oz)	0–10	3
Cider	½ cup (4 fl oz)	60	3
Miso	1 glass (6 fl oz)	283	2
Tofu	1 slice (100 g)	77	2
Apricot	4 small	67	2
Lemon juice	½ cup (4 oz)	30	2
Tempeh	½ cup	160	2
Red cabbage	½ cup	10	2
Artichoke	1 small	60	2
Leek	½ cup	27	2
Cherry tomato	6	18	2
Grape (white)	17	60	2
Soy milk	1 cup (8 fl oz)	115	2
Peach	1	40	2
Broccoli	3 spears	30	1
Potato	1	145	1
Celery	1 cup	16	1
Beans (green or white)	½ cup	20–100	1
Raspberry	¾ cup	48	1
Parsley	¼ cup	50	1
Red pepper	1 small	20	1
Tomato	1 small	20	1

*Source: USDA National Nutrient Database.

Optimize Your Food Choices

Additional aspects of the Xeno Diet include following the 80-20 rule (80 percent plant based and 20 percent animal based), focusing on foods low on the food chain, avoiding refined flour and breads, limiting processed foods, and eating natural and organic foods where possible. Table 11 lists foods to choose and foods to limit in order to help guide you to make healthy choices the xeno way. The sample menus and recipes that follow these principles demonstrate how simple and satisfying it can be to plan your Xeno Diet.

TABLE 11

Food Group	Foods to Choose	Foods to Limit
Fruits and vegetables	All fresh fruits and vegetables, preferably organic—the higher the xeno score, the better (see table 10) Frozen fruits and vegetables (but fresh is preferable) Freeze-dried fruits and vegetables Freshly squeezed 100 percent fruit and vegetable juice	Any canned, dried, or prepackaged fruits and vegetables Processed fruit juice
Grains	Whole grain or rice-based bread, cereals, bagels, crackers, pasta, pastina, couscous (at least 2 grams of fiber per serving) Brown rice Quinoa Basmati rice Rice cakes Amaranth Millet Buckwheat	White bread, pasta, rice, crackers, etc. (made with refined flour and less than 2 grams of fiber per serving)
Dairy	Low-fat milk, cheese, yogurt (organic, soy, and rice based are preferable)	Any dairy product that is not low fat Processed cheese and spreads

(continued)

Food Group	Foods to Choose	Foods to Limit
Meat/meat substitutes	Fish Skinless poultry Extra-lean beef All nuts except flavored or coated nuts All beans Tofu and soybean products Nut butters such as all-natural peanut butter, almond butter, and cashew butter (without hydrogenated oils, preservatives, sweeteners, or additives) All seeds (examples: flaxseed, pumpkin seeds, sesame seeds, sunflower seeds)	Lunch meat; hot dogs; sausage, bacon; smoked meat; breaded or fried meat; prepackaged, canned, or processed meat; egg substitutes; processed nut butters that contain hydrogenated oils, preservatives, sweeteners, or additives
Fats and oils	Olive oil, sesame oil, or flax oil Ghee (clarified butter)	Margarine, butter, vegetable oil, any trans fat (hydrogenated oil) (check labels of snack foods), fried foods
Other	Decaffeinated herbal tea, green tea, and black tea	Sugar (including sucrose, dextrose, and brown sugar), high-fructose corn syrup
Condiments	Pepper Garlic Lemon Any fresh herbs All natural spices Preservative-free soy sauce Small amounts of mustard or vinegar	Anything with artificial preservatives, flavorings, and colorings Anything with sulfites, nitrates, BHA, BHT, MSG Artificial sweeteners

Your Sample Xeno Diet Plan

Now you're on your way to planning your Xeno Diet. I have included a week's worth of menus. Since there is no such thing as a one-size-fits-all plan, these menus were developed to provide you with examples. You may choose to follow the menus just as they are or use them along with the other food lists and recipes as guidelines for planning your day. On average, the menus supply approximately 1,800 calories per day. Most people need at least that amount to maintain a healthy weight. Depending upon your age, gender, lifestyle, and nutritional goals, you may need more or fewer calories. Work with a health-care professional to define your nutritional requirements and to adjust the diet to your needs.

In general, the menus will help maximize your xeno score (polyphenol intake) and ensure adequate nutrient intake while limiting the fats, toxins, and chemicals consumed. This diet plan is also heart healthy, appropriate for blood glucose control, anti-inflammatory, and oriented toward weight management, hunger management, and overall health. The menus also incorporate some of the recipes found in the recipe section of this chapter.

Day 1

Xeno Score: 20

Breakfast
$\frac{1}{2}$ whole wheat bagel topped with 2 tablespoons light yogurt
$\frac{3}{4}$ cup raspberries
$\frac{1}{2}$ cup freshly squeezed orange juice
6 ounces decaffeinated green tea with 1 teaspoon fresh lemon
   juice

Lunch

Salmon Salad

4 ounces baked or grilled salmon	$\frac{1}{4}$ yellow onion
2 cups romaine lettuce	$\frac{1}{2}$ cup celery
$\frac{1}{4}$ sliced cucumber	$\frac{1}{4}$ cup almond slivers
$\frac{1}{4}$ tomato	

Homemade Dressing

2 tablespoons balsamic vinegar   1 tablespoon water
1 tablespoon olive oil

Season to taste with fresh herbs and/or natural seasonings.

Water

Snack
3 pieces celery filled with 1 tablespoon all-natural,
   sugar-free peanut butter
Water

Dinner
5 ounces baked boneless, skinless chicken breast marinated
   and cooked in light dressing (consider homemade dressing
   recipe from lunch)
½ cup brown rice with 1 teaspoon light olive oil spread
1 cup steamed asparagus drizzled with 1 teaspoon olive oil
   and 2 teaspoons lemon juice; seasoned to taste
Water
Red wine (1–2 glasses)

Dessert
Strawbrosia Parfait (see recipe, page 262)
Water

Day 2

Xeno Score: 32

Breakfast
Banana Berry Jumble (see recipe, page 236)
1 piece whole wheat toast with 1 teaspoon preserves
6 ounces green tea with 1 tsp fresh lemon juice

Lunch

Bean Burrito

½ cup black beans
¼ cup chopped onion
¼ cup chopped tomato

1 tablespoon chopped cilantro
2 tablespoons low-fat shredded
   soy cheese

Wrap in an 8-inch organic whole wheat tortilla.

1 cup soy yogurt
¾ cup blueberries
Water

Dinner

4 ounces lean roast beef cooked with garlic, pepper, and
   natural spices
½ organic red potato, brushed with olive oil, parsley, and
   garlic, and baked
5 baby carrots, cooked
Water
Red wine (1–2 glasses)

Dessert

12 cherries
2 pieces dark chocolate
1 cup soy milk

Day 3

Xeno Score: 24

Breakfast

Black and Blue Berry Smoothie (see recipe, page 232)
2 slices toast topped with 2 tablespoons all-natural, sugar-free
   peanut butter
8 ounces green tea

Lunch
Colorful Edamame Salad (see recipe, page 252)
2 small plums
10 whole wheat crackers
1 cup soy yogurt
Water

Dinner
4 ounces grilled whitefish with lemon juice and 1 teaspoon
    olive oil; season to taste
1 cup steamed broccoli with 1 tablespoon low-fat shredded
    cheese
³/₄ cup quinoa or brown rice topped with light olive oil spread
Water
Red wine (1–2 glasses)

Snack
1 tomato
3 slices fresh mozzarella cheese
Basil seasoning
Water

Day 4

Xeno Score: 24

Breakfast
Broccoli Frittata (see recipe, page 238)
6 ounces green tea with 1 teaspoon fresh lemon juice

Lunch

Grilled Chicken Wrap

5 oz grilled, skinless chicken	1 tablespoon low-fat shredded cheese
¹/₂ chopped onion and tomato	1 teaspoon brown all-natural mustard

Wrap in an 8-inch organic whole wheat tortilla.

1 cup fat-free soy milk
Water

Snack
⅓ cup peanuts
4 baby carrots
Water

Dinner
Black Bean, Pasta, and Artichoke Heart Medley (see recipe,
    page 244)
Tossed salad with oil and vinegar
1 slice whole wheat bread topped with garlic and
    1 teaspoon olive oil
Water
Red wine (1–2 glasses)

Dessert
Spicy Apple-filled Squash (see recipe, page 264)

Day 5

Xeno Score: 33

Breakfast
1 cup puffed rice cereal with ½ cup fat-free soy milk,
    and 1 sliced banana
6 ounces green tea with 1 teaspoon fresh lemon juice
Water

Lunch
Apple Tuna Sandwich (see recipe, page 242)
1 cup light yogurt
1 pear

Snack
6 rice bran crackers
2 slices low-fat cheese (preferably soy cheese)
Water

Dinner
Chicken Broccoli Stir-fry (see recipe, page 246)
Water
Red wine (1–2 glasses)

Dessert
Watermelon Blueberry Banana Split (see recipe, page 266)
1 cup green tea

Day 6

Xeno Score: 38

Breakfast
1 orange
2 plain rice cakes topped with 2 tablespoons all-natural, sugar-
   free almond butter
1 cup green tea
Water

Lunch
Stuffed Eggplant (see recipe, page 248)
Fruit Salad (see recipe, page 254)
Water

Snack
2 dark chocolate–covered coffee beans
1¼ cups strawberries
Water

Dinner

Lettuce Tacos

3 iceberg lettuce wedges (use as taco shells)

FILLING
$1/3$ lb lean ground turkey with all-natural seasonings
4 tablespoons homemade salsa (tomatoes, onions, cilantro, lime juice, and garlic)
2 tablespoons low-fat shredded soy cheese
$1/3$ avocado

Red wine (1–2 glasses)

Dessert
Berry Blast Smoothie (see recipe, page 234)

Day 7

Xeno Score: 26

Breakfast
1 cup oatmeal
17 grapes
1 cup green tea

Lunch
Artichoke and Roasted Red Pepper Salad with Roasted Pepper Dressing (see recipe, page 250)
1 slice whole wheat bread
Water

Snack
1 kiwifruit
1 small granola bar

Dinner

6 ounces fish (salmon, whitefish, or flounder) cooked with
1 teaspoon olive oil, garlic, and 2 teaspoons lemon juice,
seasoned to taste

1 cup broccoli topped with 2 tablespoons low-fat shredded
cheese, melted

½ cup cooked couscous with 1 teaspoon olive oil spread

1 cup fat-free soy milk

Water

Red wine (1–2 glasses)

Snack

20 organic blue corn tortilla chips

Tomatillo Salsa (see recipe, page 260)

Water

Xeno Antiaging Recipes

XENO SMOOTHIES

Black and Blue Berry Smoothie
Xeno score per serving: 8

Source: Centers for Disease Control and Prevention (CDC)

4 SERVINGS, 1 CUP OF FRUIT PER SERVING

2 cups blackberries

2 cups blueberries

1 cup fat-free plain yogurt

1 cup fat-free milk

1 teaspoon vanilla extract

2 cups ice

Place all ingredients into blender and blend until smooth. Serve immediately.

Nutrition Facts

Black and Blue Berry Smoothie
Serving Size ¼ of recipe

Amount Per Serving

Calories 120	Calories from Fat 5

	% Daily Value (DV)*
Total Fat 1g	1%
Saturated Fat 0g	0%
Trans Fat 0g	0%
Cholesterol 2mg	0%
Sodium 70mg	3%
Total Carbohydrate 26g	8%
Dietary Fiber 5g	20%
Sugars 17g	

Protein 6g	

Vitamin A	10%
Vitamin C	40%
Calcium	15%
Iron	4%

*Percent Daily Values are based on a 2,000 calorie diet.

Diabetic Exchange*

Fruit: 1
Vegetables: 0
Meat: 0
Milk: 1
Fat: 0
Carbs: 0
Other: 0

*Diabetic exchanges are calculated based on the American Diabetes Association Exchange System. This site rounds exchanges up or down to equal whole numbers. Therefore partial exchanges are not included.

Berry Blast Smoothie
Xeno score per serving: 8

Source: Centers for Disease Control and Prevention (CDC)

8 SERVINGS, 1 CUP FRUIT PER SERVING

2 cups blueberries

2 cups raspberries

2 cups strawberries

2 cups blackberries

1 cup 100% cran-raspberry juice

1 cup low-fat blueberry yogurt

2 cups ice

Place all items into blender and blend until smooth. Serve immediately.

Nutrition Facts

Berry Blast Smoothie
Serving Size ⅛ of recipe

Amount Per Serving

Calories 100	Calories from Fat 5

	% Daily Value (DV)*
Total Fat 1g	1%
Saturated Fat 0g	0%
Trans Fat 0g	0%
Cholesterol 0mg	0%
Sodium 20mg	1%
Total Carbohydrate 25g	8%
Dietary Fiber 6g	24%
Sugars 15g	
Protein 2g	
Vitamin A	2%
Vitamin C	70%
Calcium	6%
Iron	4%

*Percent Daily Values are based on a 2,000 calorie diet.

Diabetic Exchange*

Fruit: 1
Vegetables: 0
Meat: 0
Milk: 0
Fat: 0
Carbs: 0
Other: 0

*Diabetic exchanges are calculated based on the American Diabetes Association Exchange System. This site rounds exchanges up or down to equal whole numbers. Therefore partial exchanges are not included.

Vegetable Connection Smoothie
Xeno score per serving: 4

Source: Centers for Disease Control and Prevention (CDC)

4 SERVINGS, 1 CUP FRUIT AND VEGETABLES PER SERVING

1 cup sliced carrots

1 cup 100% apple juice

1 cup applesauce

1 cup sliced celery

½ cup sliced green peppers

½ cup fat-free milk

2 cups ice

Place all ingredients into blender and blend until smooth. Serve immediately.

Nutrition Facts

Vegetable Connection Smoothie
Serving Size ¼ of recipe

Amount Per Serving

Calories 90	Calories from Fat 0

	% Daily Value (DV)*
Total Fat 0g	**0%**
Saturated Fat 0g	**0%**
Trans Fat 0g	**0%**
Cholesterol 0mg	**0%**
Sodium 65mg	**3%**
Total Carbohydrate 20g	**7%**
Dietary Fiber 2g	**8%**
Sugars 17g	

Protein 2g

Vitamin A	**110%**
Vitamin C	**20%**
Calcium	**8%**
Iron	**2%**

*Percent Daily Values are based on a 2,000 calorie diet.

Diabetic Exchange*

Fruit: 1
Vegetables: 1
Meat: 0
Milk: 0
Fat: 0
Carbs: 0
Other: 0

*Diabetic exchanges are calculated based on the American Diabetes Association Exchange System. This site rounds exchanges up or down to equal whole numbers. Therefore partial exchanges are not included.

XENO BREAKFAST IDEAS

Banana Berry Jumble
Xeno score per serving: 4

Source: Centers for Disease Control and Prevention (CDC)

2 SERVINGS, ¾ CUP FRUIT PER SERVING

1 large banana, halved and cut into ½-inch pieces
¾ cup fresh or frozen cranberries
¼ cup oats
½ teaspoon nutmeg

Combine all ingredients in a large nonstick skillet. Cook on medium-high heat just until cranberries begin to soften, stirring occasionally. Remove from heat; cool slightly. Spoon into bowls and top with low-fat whipped topping, fat-free sour cream, or low-fat frozen yogurt, if desired.

Nutrition Facts

Banana Berry Jumble
Serving Size ½ of recipe

Amount Per Serving

Calories 160   Calories from Fat 15

	% Daily Value (DV)*
Total Fat 2g	**3%**
Saturated Fat 0g	**0%**
Trans Fat 0g	**0%**
Cholesterol 0mg	**0%**
Sodium 0mg	**0%**
Total Carbohydrate 33g	**11%**
Dietary Fiber 6g	**24%**
Sugars 10g	
Protein 4g	
Vitamin A	**2%**
Vitamin C	**20%**
Calcium	**2%**
Iron	**6%**

*Percent Daily Values are based on a 2,000 calorie diet.

Diabetic Exchange*

Fruit: 1
Vegetables: 0
Meat: 0
Milk: 0
Fat: 0
Carbs: 1
Other: 0

*Diabetic exchanges are calculated based on the American Diabetes Association Exchange System. This site rounds exchanges up or down to equal whole numbers. Therefore partial exchanges are not included.

Broccoli Frittata
Xeno score per serving: 4

Source: Centers for Disease Control and Prevention (CDC)

4 SERVINGS, ½ CUP VEGETABLES PER SERVING

½ cup nonfat cottage cheese

2 cups egg whites

1 large onion, diced

2 cups frozen chopped broccoli

1 teaspoon olive oil

½ teaspoon dried dill

2 teaspoons butter

Mix cottage cheese and egg whites together; set aside. In large nonstick frying pan over medium heat, sauté onion in oil for 5 minutes or until soft. Add broccoli and dill; sauté for 5 minutes or until broccoli mixture softens. Set vegetable aside.

Wipe out frying pan. Add 1 teaspoon butter and swirl the pan to distribute it. Add half of the vegetable mixture, and then add half of the egg mixture; lift and rotate pan so that eggs are evenly distributed. As eggs set around the edges, lift them to allow uncooked portions to flow underneath. Turn heat to low, cover the pan, and cook until top is set. Invert onto a serving plate and cut into wedges. Repeat with remaining 1 teaspoon butter, vegetable mixture, and egg mixture.

Nutrition Facts

Broccoli Frittata
Serving Size ¼ of recipe

Amount Per Serving

Calories 150   Calories from Fat 30

	% Daily Value (DV)*
Total Fat 3g	**5%**
Saturated Fat 0g	**0%**
Trans Fat 0g	**0%**
Cholesterol 0mg	**0%**
Sodium 390mg	**16%**
Total Carbohydrate 12g	**4%**
Dietary Fiber 3g	**12%**
Sugars 6g	
Protein 19g	
Vitamin A	**30%**
Vitamin C	**60%**
Calcium	**10%**
Iron	**15%**

*Percent Daily Values are based on a 2,000 calorie diet.

Diabetic Exchange*

Fruit: 0
Vegetables: 1
Meat: 2
Milk: 0
Fat: 1
Carbs: 0
Other: 0

*Diabetic exchanges are calculated based on the American Diabetes Association Exchange System. This site rounds exchanges up or down to equal whole numbers. Therefore partial exchanges are not included.

Golden Apple Oatmeal
Xeno score per serving: 3

Source: Centers for Disease Control and Prevention (CDC)

1 SERVING, ½ CUP FRUIT PER SERVING

1 Golden Delicious apple, diced
⅓ cup apple juice
⅓ cup water
Dash of cinnamon
Dash of nutmeg
⅓ cup quick-cook rolled oats, uncooked

Combine apples, juice, water, and seasonings in a saucepan; bring to a boil. Stir in rolled oats; cook 1 minute. Cover and let stand several minutes before serving.

Nutrition Facts

Golden Apple Oatmeal
Serving Size 1 recipe

Amount Per Serving

Calories 200 | Calories from Fat 20

	% Daily Value (DV)*
Total Fat 2g	**3%**
Saturated Fat 0g	**0%**
Trans Fat 0g	**0%**
Cholesterol 0mg	**0%**
Sodium 300mg	**13%**
Total Carbohydrate 45g	**15%**
Dietary Fiber 6g	**24%**
Sugars 23g	
Protein 4g	

Vitamin A	**2%**
Vitamin C	**10%**
Calcium	**2%**
Iron	**8%**

*Percent Daily Values are based on a 2,000 calorie diet.

Diabetic Exchange*

Fruit: 2
Vegetables: 0
Meat: 0
Milk: 0
Fat: 0
Carbs: 1
Other: 0

*Diabetic exchanges are calculated based on the American Diabetes Association Exchange System. This site rounds exchanges up or down to equal whole numbers. Therefore partial exchanges are not included.

XENO ENTRÉES

Apple Tuna Sandwich
Xeno score per serving: 4

Source: Centers for Disease Control and Prevention (CDC)

3 SERVINGS, ³/₄ CUP FRUIT PER SERVING

Two 6-ounce cans unsalted tuna in water, drained
1 medium apple, chopped
1 celery stalk, peeled and chopped
¼ cup low-fat vanilla yogurt
1 teaspoon prepared mustard
1 teaspoon honey
6 slices whole wheat bread
6 lettuce leaves
6 slices tomato

Combine and mix the tuna, apple, celery, yogurt, mustard, and honey. Spread ½ cup of the mixture on three bread slices. Top each slice of bread with lettuce, tomato, and remaining bread. Cut sandwiches in half or as desired.

Nutrition Facts

Apple Tuna Sandwich
Serving Size 1 sandwich

Amount Per Serving

Calories 330   Calories from Fat 30

	% Daily Value (DV)*
Total Fat 4g	**5%**
Saturated Fat 1g	**5%**
Trans Fat 0g	**0%**
Cholesterol 35mg	**12%**
Sodium 370mg	**15%**
Total Carbohydrate 37g	**12%**
Dietary Fiber 6g	**24%**
Sugars 14g	
Protein 38g	
Vitamin A	**40%**
Vitamin C	**20%**
Calcium	**15%**
Iron	**20%**

*Percent Daily Values are based on a 2,000 calorie diet.

Diabetic Exchange*

Fruit: 0
Vegetables: 0
Meat: 4
Milk: 0
Fat: 0
Carbs: 2
Other: 0

*Diabetic exchanges are calculated based on the American Diabetes Association Exchange System. This site rounds exchanges up or down to equal whole numbers. Therefore partial exchanges are not included.

Black Bean, Pasta, and Artichoke Heart Medley

Xeno score per serving: 4

Source: Centers for Disease Control and Prevention (CDC)

12 SERVINGS, ½ CUP VEGETABLES PER SERVING

1 tablespoon olive oil
1 cup sliced green onions
½ teaspoon oregano
½ teaspoon basil
¼ teaspoon salt
⅛ teaspoon black pepper
⅛ teaspoon cayenne pepper
1 garlic clove, minced
Two 14½-ounce cans whole tomatoes (no added salt),
    undrained and chopped
One 15-ounce can black beans, rinsed and drained
4 cups hot, cooked pasta (any shape)
One 14-ounce can artichoke hearts, drained and quartered

Heat oil in a large nonstick skillet over medium heat. Add green onions
and sauté 5 minutes. Add oregano, basil, salt, peppers, garlic, and
tomatoes; cover and simmer 10 minutes. Add beans; cover and simmer
an additional 5 minutes. Combine bean mixture, hot cooked pasta,
and artichoke hearts in a large bowl. Toss well. Serve warm or at room
temperature.

Nutrition Facts

Black Bean, Pasta, and Artichoke Heart
Medley
Serving Size $1/12$ of recipe

Amount Per Serving

Calories 120   Calories from Fat 15

	% Daily Value (DV)*
Total Fat 2g	3%
Saturated Fat 0g	0%
Trans Fat 0g	0%
Cholesterol 0mg	0%
Sodium 330mg	14%
Total Carbohydrate 21g	7%
Dietary Fiber 3g	12%
Sugars 2g	

Protein 5g

Vitamin A	4%
Vitamin C	15%
Calcium	4%
Iron	15%

*Percent Daily Values are based on a 2,000 calorie diet.

Diabetic Exchange*

Fruit: 0
Vegetables: 1
Meat: 0
Milk: 0
Fat: 0
Carbs: 1
Other: 0

*Diabetic exchanges are calculated based on the American Diabetes Association Exchange System. This site rounds exchanges up or down to equal whole numbers. Therefore partial exchanges are not included.

Chicken Broccoli Stir-fry
Xeno score per serving: 5

Source: Centers for Disease Control and Prevention (CDC)

4 SERVINGS, 1 CUP OF VEGETABLES PER SERVING

1/3 cup orange juice

1 tablespoon low-sodium soy sauce

1 tablespoon Szechuan sauce

2 teaspoons cornstarch

1 tablespoon canola oil

1 pound boneless chicken breast, cut into 1-inch cubes

2 cups shredded cabbage

2 cups of frozen broccoli florets

1 6-ounce package of frozen snow peas

2 cups of cooked brown rice

1 tablespoon sesame seeds (optional)

Mix orange juice, soy sauce, Szechuan sauce, and cornstarch in a small bowl. Set aside. Heat oil in wok and add chicken. Stir-fry for about 5 to 7 minutes. Add cabbage, broccoli, snow peas, and sauce mixture. Cook for about 5 minutes until vegetables are heated through. Serve over brown rice. Sprinkle with sesame seeds.

Nutrition Facts

Chicken Broccoli Stir-fry
Serving Size ¼ of recipe

Amount Per Serving

Calories 340   Calories from Fat 70

	% Daily Value (DV)*
Total Fat 8g	**12%**
Saturated Fat 2g	**8%**
Trans Fat 0g	**0%**
Cholesterol 65mg	**22%**
Sodium 240mg	**10%**
Total Carbohydrate 35g	**12%**
Dietary Fiber 5g	**20%**
Sugars 5g	
Protein 28g	
Vitamin A	**4%**
Vitamin C	**70%**
Calcium	**8%**
Iron	**15%**

*Percent Daily Values are based on a 2,000 calorie diet.

Diabetic Exchange*

Fruit: 0
Vegetables: 1
Meat: 3
Milk: 0
Fat: 1
Carbs: 1
Other: 0

*Diabetic exchanges are calculated based on the American Diabetes Association Exchange System. This site rounds exchanges up or down to equal whole numbers. Therefore partial exchanges are not included.

Stuffed Eggplant
Xeno score per serving: 10

Source: Centers for Disease Control and Prevention (CDC)

4 SERVINGS, 2 CUPS OF VEGETABLES PER SERVING

2 eggplants
Vegetable cooking spray
2 diced tomatoes
$\frac{1}{2}$ cup diced green bell pepper
$\frac{1}{2}$ cup diced onion
$\frac{1}{3}$ cup diced celery
$1\frac{1}{2}$ cups bread crumbs
2 tablespoons fresh minced parsley
2 tablespoons fat-free Parmesan cheese

Preheat oven to 350°F. Cut eggplants in half lengthwise. Scoop out and save the flesh, leaving the shells $\frac{3}{8}$ inch thick. If necessary, trim a small piece off the bottom of each shell so it won't tip over. Set aside.

Coat large skillet with vegetable cooking spray. Chop up reserved eggplant and add to skillet. Add tomato, bell pepper, onion, and celery. Place skillet over medium heat; cover and cook about 5 minutes, until vegetables are tender. Remove skillet from heat. Stir in bread crumbs and parsley. Spoon mixture into the hollow eggplant shells.

Arrange stuffed shells in a shallow baking dish coated with vegetable spray. Sprinkle $1\frac{1}{2}$ teaspoon Parmesan on top of each shell. Bake for 25 minutes, until filling is heated through and top is golden brown.

Nutrition Facts

Stuffed Eggplant
Serving Size ¼ of recipe

Amount Per Serving

Calories 270   Calories from Fat 30

	% Daily Value (DV)*
Total Fat 4g	**5%**
Saturated Fat 0g	**0%**
Trans Fat 0g	**0%**
Cholesterol 0mg	**0%**
Sodium 360mg	**15%**
Total Carbohydrate 51g	**17%**
Dietary Fiber 13g	**48%**
Sugars 11g	
Protein 11g	
Vitamin A	**20%**
Vitamin C	**50%**
Calcium	**10%**
Iron	**20%**

*Percent Daily Values are based on a 2,000 calorie diet.

Diabetic Exchange*

Fruit: 0
Vegetables: 4
Meat: 0
Milk: 0
Fat: 0
Carbs: 2
Other: 0

*Diabetic exchanges are calculated based on the American Diabetes Association Exchange System. This site rounds exchanges up or down to equal whole numbers. Therefore partial exchanges are not included.

XENO SIDES AND SALADS

Artichoke and Roasted Red Pepper Salad with Roasted Pepper Dressing
Xeno score per serving: 4

Source: Centers for Disease Control and Prevention (CDC)

8 SERVINGS, 1½ CUPS OF VEGETABLE PER SERVING

8 medium artichokes, prepared and cooked as directed
    for whole artichokes
3 red bell peppers
Lettuce leaves
½ cup sliced red onion
½ cup sliced black olives

DRESSING
1 bell pepper (roasted), reserved from salad preparation
⅓ cup balsamic vinegar
¼ cup white wine or cider vinegar
2 cloves garlic, minced
1 tablespoon chopped fresh basil or 1 teaspoon crushed dried basil
1 teaspoon chopped fresh rosemary or ½ teaspoon crushed
    dried rosemary
1 teaspoon sugar

Halve artichokes lengthwise; scoop out center petals and fuzzy centers.
Remove outer leaves and reserve to garnish salad, or to use for snacks
another time. Trim out hearts and slice thinly. Cover and set aside. Place
whole bell peppers under preheated broiler; broil under high heat until
charred on all sides, turning frequently with tongs. Remove from oven;
place in a paper bag for 15 minutes to steam skins. Trim off stems of
peppers; remove seeds and ribs. Strip off skins; slice peppers into juli-
enne strips. Reserve ¼ of the bell pepper strips to prepare dressing.

    To assemble salads, arrange lettuce leaves on 8 salad plates.
Arrange sliced artichoke hearts, remaining bell pepper strips, red onion,

and olive slices on lettuce. Garnish with a couple of cooked artichoke leaves, if desired.

DRESSING

For dressing, in blender or food processor container place reserved bell pepper strips, vinegars, garlic, basil, rosemary, and sugar. Cover and process until well blended and nearly smooth. Spoon dressing over salads.

Nutrition Facts

Artichoke and Roasted Red Pepper Salad
with Roasted Pepper Dressing
Serving Size ⅛ recipe

Amount Per Serving

Calories 110   Calories from Fat 10

	% Daily Value (DV)*
Total Fat 2g	2%
Saturated Fat 0g	0%
Trans Fat 0g	0%
Cholesterol 0mg	0%
Sodium 200mg	8%
Total Carbohydrate 22g	7%
Dietary Fiber 9g	36%
Sugars 8g	
Protein 5g	
Vitamin A	70%
Vitamin C	270%
Calcium	8%
Iron	15%

*Percent Daily Values are based on a 2,000 calorie diet.

Diabetic Exchange*

Fruit: 0
Vegetables: 4
Meat: 0
Milk: 0
Fat: 0
Carbs: 0
Other: 0

*Diabetic exchanges are calculated based on the American Diabetes Association Exchange System. This site rounds exchanges up or down to equal whole numbers. Therefore partial exchanges are not included.

Colorful Edamame Salad
Xeno score per serving: 6

Source: Centers for Disease Control and Prevention (CDC)

4 SERVINGS, 2 CUPS OF VEGETABLES PER SERVING

1½ cups shelled edamame

4 cups romaine lettuce, washed

1 cup shredded carrots

2 cups cherry tomatoes

1 cup sliced cucumber

½ cup chopped red onion

To cook edamame, bring 3 cups water to a boil. Add shelled edamame and cook 4 minutes. Drain and rinse with cold running water to cool. Prepare all other ingredients and combine with the edamame in a large salad bowl. If desired, toss with a low-fat or nonfat dressing of your choice.

Note: The dressing is not included in the nutritional analysis.

Nutrition Facts

Colorful Edamame Salad
Serving Size ¼ recipe

Amount Per Serving

Calories 120	Calories from Fat 20

	% Daily Value (DV)*
Total Fat 3g	**4%**
Saturated Fat 0g	**0%**
Trans Fat 0g	**0%**
Cholesterol 0mg	**0%**
Sodium 80mg	**3%**
Total Carbohydrate 17g	**6%**
Dietary Fiber 4g	**16%**
Sugars 7g	
Protein 9g	

Vitamin A	**150%**
Vitamin C	**45%**
Calcium	**10%**
Iron	**10%**

*Percent Daily Values are based on a 2,000 calorie diet.

Diabetic Exchange*

Fruit: 0
Vegetables: 2
Meat: 1
Milk: 0
Fat: 0
Carbs: 0
Other: 0

*Diabetic exchanges are calculated based on the American Diabetes Association Exchange System. This site rounds exchanges up or down to equal whole numbers. Therefore partial exchanges are not included.

Fruit Salad

Xeno score per serving: 5

Source: Centers for Disease Control and Prevention (CDC)

4 SERVINGS, ½ CUP OF FRUIT PER SERVING

½ cup sliced banana   ½ cup grapes
½ cup chopped apple   ½ cup orange juice
½ cup chopped papaya

In a medium bowl, mix all ingredients. Serve.

Nutrition Facts

Fruit Salad
Serving Size ¼ of recipe

Amount Per Serving

Calories 60	Calories from Fat 0

	% Daily Value (DV)*
Total Fat 0g	0%
Saturated Fat 0g	0%
Trans Fat 0g	0%
Cholesterol 0mg	0%
Sodium 0mg	0%
Total Carbohydrate 15g	5%
Dietary Fiber 1g	4%
Sugars 11g	

Protein 1g

Vitamin A	6%
Vitamin C	50%
Calcium	2%
Iron	2%

*Percent Daily Values are based on a 2,000 calorie diet.

Diabetic Exchange*

Fruit: 1
Vegetables: 0
Meat: 0
Milk: 0
Fat: 0
Carbs: 0
Other: 0

*Diabetic exchanges are calculated based on the American Diabetes Association Exchange System. This site rounds exchanges up or down to equal whole numbers. Therefore partial exchanges are not included.

XENO DIPS, SPREADS, SALSAS

Baba Ghanoush (Eggplant Dip)
Xeno score per serving: 7

Source: Centers for Disease Control and Prevention (CDC)

8 SERVINGS, ³/₄ CUP OF VEGETABLES PER SERVING

2 large eggplants (1¼ pounds)
2 tablespoons tahini
4 cloves garlic, peeled and crushed
½ cup diced onion
1 cup chopped tomato
3 tablespoons fresh lemon juice or more to taste
4 tablespoons cold water
¼ teaspoon salt
⅛ teaspoon freshly ground black pepper
½ teaspoon olive oil
Parsley sprigs to garnish (optional)

Pierce the eggplants in several places with a toothpick or fork. Wrap each eggplant in aluminum foil and place on a gas grill or in the oven at 500°F. Cook until the eggplants collapse and begin to release a lot of steam, about 10 to 15 minutes. Remove the foil and place the eggplants in a bowl of cold water. Peel while eggplants are still hot and allow them to drain in a colander until cool. Squeeze pulp to remove any bitter juices and mash the eggplant to a puree.

In a food processor, mix tahini, garlic, onion, tomato, lemon juice, and water until mixture is concentrated. With the blender running, add the peeled eggplant, salt, pepper, and olive oil. Serve in a shallow dish and garnish with black pepper, tomatoes, and parsley.

Nutrition Facts

Baba Ghanoush (Eggplant Dip)
Serving Size ⅛ of recipe

Amount Per Serving

Calories 70	Calories from Fat 25

	% Daily Value (DV)*
Total Fat 3g	**4%**
Saturated Fat 0g	**0%**
Trans Fat 0g	**0%**
Cholesterol 0 mg	**0%**
Sodium 80mg	**3%**
Total Carbohydrate 11g	**4%**
Dietary Fiber 5g	**20%**
Sugars 4g	

Protein 2g	

Vitamin A	**4%**
Vitamin C	**15%**
Calcium	**4%**
Iron	**4%**

*Percent Daily Values are based on a 2,000 calorie diet.

Diabetic Exchange*

Fruit: 0
Vegetables: 2
Meat: 0
Milk: 0
Fat: 0
Carbs: 0
Other: 0

*Diabetic exchanges are calculated based on the American Diabetes Association Exchange System. This site rounds exchanges up or down to equal whole numbers. Therefore partial exchanges are not included.

Fresh Northwest Cherry Salsa
Xeno score per serving: 4

Source: Centers for Disease Control and Prevention (CDC)

4 SERVINGS, ½ CUP OF FRUIT AND VEGETABLES PER SERVING

2 cups pitted fresh or frozen sweet cherries
⅓ cup chopped fresh basil
⅓ cup finely chopped green bell pepper
2 teaspoons lemon juice
½ teaspoon Worcestershire sauce
½ teaspoon grated lemon peel
¼ teaspoon salt
Dash of bottled hot pepper sauce

Chop cherries in food processor or with a knife. Combine all ingredients; mix well. Refrigerate at least 1 hour.

Nutrition Facts

Fresh Northwest Cherry Salsa
Serving Size 1/4 recipe

Amount Per Serving

Calories 50   Calories from Fat 0

	% Daily Value (DV)*
Total Fat 0g	0%
Saturated Fat 0g	0%
Trans Fat 0g	0%
Cholesterol 0mg	0%
Sodium 160mg	7%
Total Carbohydrate 13g	4%
Dietary Fiber 2g	8%
Sugars 10g	
Protein 1g	
Vitamin A	6%
Vitamin C	30%
Calcium	2%
Iron	2%

*Percent Daily Values are based on a 2,000 calorie diet.

Diabetic Exchange*

Fruit: 1
Vegetables: 0
Meat: 0
Milk: 0
Fat: 0
Carbs: 0
Other: 0

*Diabetic exchanges are calculated based on the American Diabetes Association Exchange System. This site rounds exchanges up or down to equal whole numbers. Therefore partial exchanges are not included.

Rhubarb Pico de Gallo

Xeno score per serving: 4

Source: Centers for Disease Control and Prevention (CDC)

8 SERVINGS, ½ CUP OF FRUIT AND VEGETABLES PER SERVING

1 cup diced rhubarb
1 cup diced tomatoes
½ teaspoon salt

1 cup diced white onions
1¼ cup chopped cilantro
Juice of ½ lime

Combine all ingredients in a bowl and mix together. Refrigerate. Serve cold.

Nutrition Facts

Rhubarb Pico de Gallo
Serving Size ⅛ recipe

Amount Per Serving

Calories 20	Calories from Fat 0

	% Daily Value (DV)*
Total Fat 0g	**0%**
Saturated Fat 0g	**0%**
Trans Fat 0g	**0%**
Cholesterol 0mg	**0%**
Sodium 150mg	**6%**
Total Carbohydrate 4g	**1%**
Dietary Fiber 1g	**4%**
Sugars 2g	

Protein 1g

Vitamin A	**8%**
Vitamin C	**15%**
Calcium	**2%**
Iron	**2%**

*Percent Daily Values are based on a 2,000 calorie diet.

Diabetic Exchange*

Fruit: 0
Vegetables: 1
Meat: 0
Milk: 0
Fat: 0
Carbs: 0
Other: 0

*Diabetic exchanges are calculated based on the American Diabetes Association Exchange System. This site rounds exchanges up or down to equal whole numbers. Therefore partial exchanges are not included.

Tomatillo Salsa
Xeno score per serving: 4

Source: Centers for Disease Control and Prevention (CDC)

4 SERVINGS, 1 CUP OF FRUIT AND VEGETABLES PER SERVING

12 tomatillos, husks removed, washed and finely chopped, or
    two 12-ounce cans tomatillos, drained and finely chopped
4 serrano chilies, finely chopped, seeded if desired
1 small white onion, finely chopped
¼ cup chopped fresh cilantro
1 clove garlic, finely chopped
Pinch of salt, optional
Pinch of sugar, optional

In a medium bowl, mix all ingredients. Season with salt and sugar,
if desired. Serve or store salsa in refrigerator for up to three days in
a covered plastic or glass container.

Nutrition Facts

Tomatillo Salsa
Serving Size ¼ of recipe, about ½ cup

Amount Per Serving

Calories 50	Calories from Fat 10

	% Daily Value (DV)*
Total Fat 1g	**2%**
Saturated Fat 0g	**0%**
Trans Fat 0g	**0%**
Cholesterol 0mg	**0%**
Sodium 75mg	**3%**
Total Carbohydrate 10g	**3%**
Dietary Fiber 3g	**12%**
Sugars 6g	
Protein 1g	
Vitamin A	**4%**
Vitamin C	**30%**
Calcium	**2%**
Iron	**4%**

*Percent Daily Values are based on a 2,000 calorie diet.

Diabetic Exchange*

Fruit: 0
Vegetables: 2
Meat: 0
Milk: 0
Fat: 0
Carbs: 0
Other: 0

*Diabetic exchanges are calculated based on the American Diabetes Association Exchange System. This site rounds exchanges up or down to equal whole numbers. Therefore partial exchanges are not included.

XENO DESSERTS

Strawbrosia Parfait
Xeno score per serving: 5

Source: Centers for Disease Control and Prevention (CDC)

6 SERVINGS, ½ CUP OF FRUIT PER SERVING

2 cups sliced strawberries

1 banana, sliced

1 orange, peeled and sliced (or 11-ounce can mandarin
orange segments)

½ cup orange juice

1 cup cubed pineapple, fresh or canned

1 cup (8-ounce carton) nonfat vanilla or lemon yogurt

¼ cup Grape-Nuts

6 mint sprigs

In a bowl, mix strawberries, banana, orange, and pineapple. Pour orange juice over fruit and toss. Refrigerate until chilled.

To prepare parfaits: Divide half of the fruit mixture equally into 6 parfait glasses. Top with heaping tablespoon of yogurt. Add remaining fruit divided equally; top with remaining yogurt. Sprinkle each parfait with Grape Nuts. Garnish each parfait with a mint sprig.

Nutrition Facts

Strawbrosia Parfaits
Serving Size ⅙ serving

Amount Per Serving

Calories 110	Calories from Fat 5

	% Daily Value (DV)*
Total Fat 0g	**0%**
Saturated Fat 0g	**0%**
Trans Fat 0g	**0%**
Cholesterol 0mg	**0%**
Sodium 60mg	**3%**
Total Carbohydrate 26g	**9%**
Dietary Fiber 3g	**12%**
Sugars 17g	

Protein 3g

Vitamin A	**4%**
Vitamin C	**100%**
Calcium	**10%**
Iron	**10%**

*Percent Daily Values are based on a 2,000 calorie diet.

Diabetic Exchange*

Fruit: 1
Vegetables: 0
Meat: 0
Milk: 0
Fat: 0
Carbs: 0
Other: 0

*Diabetic exchanges are calculated based on the American Diabetes Association Exchange System. This site rounds exchanges up or down to equal whole numbers. Therefore partial exchanges are not included.

Spicy Apple-filled Squash
Xeno score per serving: 4

Source: Centers for Disease Control and Prevention (CDC)

4 SERVINGS, ½ CUP OF FRUIT AND VEGETABLES PER SERVING

1 acorn squash (about 1 pound)
1 golden delicious apple, peeled, cored, and sliced
2 teaspoons reduced-fat margarine, melted
2 teaspoons brown sugar
⅛ teaspoon cinnamon
⅛ teaspoon nutmeg
Dash ground cloves

Heat oven to 350°F. Grease a 1-quart baking dish. Halve squash and re-move seeds; cut into quarters. Place quarters skin side up in dish and cover; bake 30 minutes. Meanwhile, in medium bowl, combine apple, margarine, brown sugar, cinnamon, nutmeg, and cloves. Turn cut sides of acorn squash up; top with apple mixture. Cover and bake 30 minutes longer or until apples are tender.

Quick microwave version: Halve and seed squash; cut into quarters. Arrange quarters cut side up in microwave-safe baking dish. Microwave on high (100 percent) 6 to 7 minutes, rotating squash halfway through cooking time. Top squash with apple mixture, cover with vented plastic wrap, and microwave on high 4 to 5 minutes, or until apples are tender.

Nutrition Facts

Spicy Apple-Filled Squash
Serving Size ¼ recipe

Amount Per Serving

Calories 80	Calories from Fat 15

	% Daily Value (DV)*
Total Fat 2g	**2%**
Saturated Fat 1g	**5%**
Trans Fat 0g	**0%**
Cholesterol 0mg	**0%**
Sodium 5mg	**0%**
Total Carbohydrate 17g	**6%**
Dietary Fiber 2g	**8%**
Sugars 7g	
Protein 1g	

Vitamin A	**10%**
Vitamin C	**25%**
Calcium	**4%**
Iron	**4%**

*Percent Daily Values are based on a 2,000 calorie diet.

Diabetic Exchange*

Fruit: 0
Vegetables: 2
Meat: 0
Milk: 0
Fat: 0
Carbs: 0
Other: 0

*Diabetic exchanges are calculated based on the American Diabetes Association Exchange System. This site rounds exchanges up or down to equal whole numbers. Therefore partial exchanges are not included.

Watermelon Blueberry Banana Split
Xeno score per serving: 5

Source: Centers for Disease Control and Prevention (CDC)

4 SERVINGS, 3 CUPS OF FRUIT PER SERVING

2 large bananas
8 watermelon "scoops"—watermelon balls created with an
   ice cream scoop
2 cups fresh blueberries
½ cup low-fat vanilla yogurt
¼ cup low-fat granola

Peel bananas and cut in half crosswise, then cut each piece in half lengthwise. For each serving, lay 2 banana pieces against the sides of a shallow dish. Place a watermelon scoop at each and of the dish. Fill the center space with blueberries. Stir yogurt until smooth and spoon over watermelon scoops. Sprinkle with granola.

Nutrition Facts

Watermelon Blueberry Banana Split
Serving Size ¼ of recipe

Amount Per Serving

Calories 160	Calories from Fat 10

	% Daily Value (DV)*
Total Fat 1g	**2%**
Saturated Fat 0g	**0%**
Trans Fat 0g	**0%**
Cholesterol 0mg	**0%**
Sodium 40mg	**2%**
Total Carbohydrate 38g	**13%**
Dietary Fiber 4g	**16%**
Sugars 23g	
Protein 4g	
Vitamin A	**6%**
Vitamin C	**25%**
Calcium	**6%**
Iron	**4%**

Percent Daily Values are based on a 2,000 calorie diet.

Diabetic Exchange*

Fruit: 2
Vegetables: 0
Meat: 0
Milk: 0
Fat: 0
Carbs: 1
Other: 0

*Diabetic exchanges are calculated based on the American Diabetes Association Exchange System. This site rounds exchanges up or down to equal whole numbers. Therefore partial exchanges are not included.

Step 4: Xeno Factors Supplements— What Kind and How Much

The vast majority of studies on weight loss, energy enhancement, and organ protection have used doses of resveratrol substantially higher than those obtainable from foods. This is not to say that food sources of resveratrol and other polyphenols are not important. Red wine, for example, is believed to impart tremendous health benefits when consumed daily in moderation. Other sources include concentrated juice extracts. These include products like the Australian extract and Naturex's Powergrape, both promising products but not yet available. Other juice products, including fruit juices like Noni, XanGo, and others that tout the health benefits of polyphenols and antioxidants, are available commercially. Nonalcoholic red grape juice and other fruit juices also can provide substantial amounts of polyphenols, but currently, only dietary supplements offer the doses of resveratrol and other polyphenols used in selected animal and human studies.

Our attention, then, must be directed to the commercially available resveratrol supplements discussed in chapter 18. The products we have most considered include those made by Resveratrol Partners (www.longevinex.com), Biotivia (www.biotivia.com), and RevGenetics (www.revegenetics.com). The sources of these products, their manufacturing procedures, their costs, and other information can be found on their respective websites. Because of the tremendous interest in this subject, there is little doubt the range of products available will be exploding. Many resveratrol products and concentrated polyphenol products, not quite yet commercially available, will soon be on the market in both capsule and drink form. The key factor in many products will be not just the amount of resveratrol or other polyphenols, but that human clinical trials are conducted on them. The optimal dosage of any of these dietary supplements or polyphenol concentrates cannot yet be confirmed based on the limited human data.

But from hundreds of laboratory studies, we believe that for a young, healthy, normally active individual, a dose in the range of 100 to 500 milligrams a day is reasonable and safe. For those over forty, a dose closer to 500 milligrams a day might be more appropriate. For athletes desiring enhanced energy and mitochondrial activity, even higher doses might be considered. As a part of my four-step xeno weight control and energy program, I personally take 250 to 500 milligrams of resveratrol per day, as well as 400 milligrams of a mixed polyphenol supplement. As noted earlier, according to an unscientific survey of those who indicated they were invested in Sirtris Pharmaceuticals, 20 percent of these individuals take more than 100,000 milligrams per day of resveratrol. No source of this product was indicated in the survey.

Please note that the statements above are not approved by the FDA and that all of this information is obtained from the current medical literature.

Chapter 20

Summing Up

*With what ease we enter into this world but with what diffi-
culty we sometimes leave it.*

—DANTE

I hope I die before I get old.

—THE WHO, 1965

In 1938 W. Somerset Maugham, the British playwright, novelist, and
physician, looked back over his life of sixty-four years and contem-
plated his most important accomplishments. He concluded in his
book *The Summing Up,* "The most important thing in life is what one
wills to create." Bringing together in this book thousands of scientific
papers and books, my visits to various laboratories, and my own personal experiences has been an exhilarating and most satisfying creative
experience. Applying the four-step longevity program and balancing
my life as well as my diet remain a work in progress.

My editor and friend Peter Guzzardi wrote in bright red in the mar-
gin of one of the innumerable drafts of this book, "What do *you* do to
balance your life and diet?" As a neurosurgeon who performs more
than 350 brain and spinal operations a year, a divorced parent with five
children, and a competitive triathlete, I have made attaining balance in
my daily life my number one priority. Each morning I consider the four
sides of my square and allocate the time that each will require. Unless I

make a conscious effort to plan ahead, review that plan daily, and pursue balance in each day's activities, I find that I slip back into chaos.

Work

With the help of my colleagues and superb staff, I am able to schedule my outpatients, my surgery, and my ongoing laboratory and writing projects into specific time slots. Although there are always exceptions and unexpected requirements, generally this approach works very well.

Physical Activity

I schedule an hour for personal fitness into each day. For me this means aerobic activity in the form of swimming, biking, or running followed by stretching and flexibility exercises six days per week. Three days a week I do resistance training with weights. When I train for a triathlon, I set aside fifteen to eighteen hours a week for that purpose.

Family Life

As a divorced parent with two daughters still in high school, I arrange to spend weekends and some evenings during the week with my children. Sports activities that involve the children and attending Pittsburgh Steelers football games (I am the Steelers' team physician) are our favorite activities. Sunday Mass together is also a priority.

Spirituality

Spiritually, I have been humbled and tested. The premature death of one son at age twenty-one in an auto accident, the incapacitation of another son from a severe birth disorder, the loss of both parents prematurely, the horrible experience of divorce, and the death and disability I have witnessed in my neurosurgical practice have, on many occasions, forced me to question the meaning and value of life itself. It is in these darkest hours that my belief in a higher power requires me to highlight what is essential and to regard everything else as secondary. Through spirit I find my life's priorities.

Though I grew up in a Roman Catholic home, I find that my philosophy and spiritual beliefs have shifted to a Christianity/Zen approach to my daily activities and problems. Over the last twenty years, I have frequently found peace, understanding, and solace at Mount Savior Monastery near Elmira, New York. There fifteen monks who have taken vows of poverty, obedience, and chastity adhere to the same beliefs, teachings, and rules set forth by Saint Benedict in the sixth century. Visitors are welcomed at no cost. Located on the top of a mountain with rolling plains and bordered by thick forests, the monastery sustains itself, as the monks raise their own organic fruits and vegetables, cultivate the fields, and raise longhorn sheep.

My brain gets its restful rewiring as I step away from my daily problems and responsibilities—even if only for a long weekend—by contemplating and meditating on what is truly important in life and experiencing how little we really need in order to survive. This experience, once or twice a year, helps me to live in the present moment, to be mindful of my activities, and to be awakened to the creative powers that lie deep within each of us.

For me there are few things more spiritual than swimming across a quiet lake in the early morning, biking down a country road, running or walking through wooded trails, or saying a prayer with a patient before entering the operating room. Although at times my life has been far out of balance, I have been like Sydney Carton in Charles Dickens's *A Tale of Two Cities:* "recalled to life" on more than one occasion by consciously attending to my square.

Balancing my diet is also a work in progress. I grew up enjoying bologna and mayonnaise sandwiches on white bread, Oreo cookies, well-marbled steaks, French fries, and gallons of Coca-Cola. When my father died suddenly at age sixty after his third heart attack, the handwriting was clearly on the wall for me. Overweight, overworked, and mentally fatigued from a relentless schedule of neurosurgery, in my late thirties I realized that nothing in my life was in balance. As I mentioned earlier, my diet changed and weight loss happened as unintended side effects of becoming physically active and working to balance my life. Now I adhere to the Xeno Diet. The 80-20 meal plan is my daily fare, with unlimited vegetables and fruits; limited sugar, flour, and salt; and balanced fats, proteins, and carbohydrates. As for liquids, I have a glass of wine or two with my evening meal, three to five cups of green tea a day, and plenty of water.

In addition to the supplements mentioned in chapter 18, I take 250 to 500 milligrams of resveratrol, 400 milligrams of a mixed polyphenol supplement, 3 grams of EPA/DHA fish oil, a multivitamin, and flaxseed, wheat germ, and walnuts with my breakfast every morning.

After having children, the most creative act we can perform is to bring balance to our lives and our diets. On the basis of my own experience, I can say with confidence that the suggestions throughout this book really work. At age sixty-eight I have more physical energy, mental awareness, and patience with my children that I ever had before. I completed my third Ironman triathlon in 2008. It is clear to me that, as with a grape, suffering through life's many adversities has made me stronger.

It is not death I fear; it is dying—and the disability related to the dying process. As a neurosurgeon, I have helped thousands of patients, but I have also futilely presided over the deaths of countless others. Many of these were afflicted with the diseases of aging—heart disease, cancer, stroke, and dementia—and in the words of the Welsh poet Dylan Thomas, they "[did] not go gentle into that good night."

As Dr. Roy Walford once said, to increase the life span and decrease the diseases of aging "has been one of humankind's oldest preoccupations; indeed, one of the great dreams of our species." Anything that would significantly contribute to that goal would be considered nearly miraculous. Business analysts now estimate that the antiaging industry generates $50 billion a year in sales. It does so by offering remedies for the *effects* of aging—creams, lotions, injections, surgery, and food supplements—under the guise of offering true antiaging. Because the industry targets only the end results of the aging process, not aging itself, you can never stop buying its products.

Is antiaging just about vanity, or does it really have a sound scientific basis? And what are the implications of adding years to our life span? Both as a doctor and as a sixty-eight-year-old, I have an intensely personal interest in the answers.

The goal of antiaging has always been at least partly about vanity, but now we're beginning to be able to intervene in the biological process of aging. With recent advances in molecular biology and the sequencing of the human genome, researchers are rapidly unraveling the genetics of aging. Studies on mold, yeast, worms, fruit flies, fish, monkeys, and now humans all confirm similar pathways of aging that evolved very early in the history of life, which give us a very real opportunity to markedly extend the life span and the health span.

Recently, Dr. Thomas Perls of Boston University School of Medicine and his team, who are studying centenarians, found a region on chromosome 4 that is linked to exceptional longevity. In this long stretch of DNA, they discovered as many as two hundred genes that may be responsible for slowing down the aging process. A genetically regulated scientific basis for life extension can no longer be questioned. But what about those of us who don't have unusual longevity in our family histories? Although genes do play a role in aging, other factors such as nutrition, exercise, lifestyle, and environment play a larger role (see figure 21). The foods that we eat or don't eat, the exercise we engage in or avoid, and the decision to use or abstain from addictive substances are also critical in determining our life span.

How much closer are we to mankind's dream of actually extending the life span? Again, the scientific studies presented in this book indicate that we are on the threshold. At the beginning of the twentieth century, life expectancy was approximately forty-five years. It is now nearly seventy-eight years and rising, thanks to a consistent food supply and the advent of antibiotics and public health measures.

So how can we maximize and increase our life span from here? Scientists now agree that the first and most accessible approach is to ad-

Genes and Lifespan

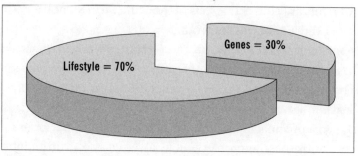

FIGURE 21 The factors that can determine longevity are partly due to your genetic makeup. But lifestyle choices, such as nutrition, exercise, and smoking—which are controlled by *you*—are the more important factors.

here to a list of five essentials: healthy diet, exercise, mental challenge, novelty in our lives, and meditation/spirituality for emotional balance. The second approach involves our genes: either we fall into that group fortunate enough to be born with good genes for longevity, or we activate such genes through healthy living and genetically bioactive compounds like those found in xeno factors. The fulfillment of the dream, therefore, appears possible, at least to some extent.

It is said that anything that sounds too good to be true usually is. Does it really make sense to think that plant-derived natural compounds can increase strength, endurance, memory, and longevity, and at the same time help us stay thin? As a skeptical scientist, I found such claims impossible to believe until David Sinclair said, "Look at the evidence yourself." Since that time, I have read extensively about the science of aging and longevity. In these pages I have attempted to simplify the extremely complex molecular biology underpinning how plants communicate with people. I have also described how plant-derived xeno factors activate genes to increase strength, endurance, and memory, and at the same time reduce inflammation, improve sugar metabolism, and increase longevity. World-renowned scientists in Boston, Baltimore, Finland, France, and Italy have all now confirmed these beneficial effects in animals.

The multibillion-dollar question is: will it work in human beings? Unfortunately, it takes many years to scientifically confirm that disease reduction and increased longevity are taking place. We *can* say that rigorous scientific studies in cell cultures, animal models, and some population studies now confirm that these plant-based substances are effective in treating and helping to prevent the diseases of aging, and that clinical studies and trials funded by the National Institutes of Health (see appendix C) and private industry are at present attempting to corroborate that these same beneficial effects hold true for humans.

After pondering this question, David Sinclair published his thoughts in the journal *Mechanisms of Aging and Development,* in an article titled, "Toward a Unified Theory of Caloric Restriction and Longevity Regulation." He wrote, "Calorie restriction provokes an active, functional response to alter metabolism. It is an ancient response that evolved to promote the survival of organisms during adversity. It also means that discoveries in simple organisms such as yeast, worms, and flies are likely to be more relevant to mammals than many had previously thought. The most practical implication is that we probably do not need to know the proximal causes of aging to develop prolonging strategies. We just need to target the longevity regulators themselves, as they will counter the causes of aging, whatever they may be." In other words, we don't need to understand the engineering principles of our car's internal combustion engine, but if we use the right fuel and provide the proper maintenance, we can make a profound difference.

The confirmation that stressed plant molecules, when ingested orally, can activate these same genetic longevity regulators makes the strongest case yet for a naturally occurring safe substance that will "counter the causes of aging, whatever they may be" in humans as in animals. The body of evidence from research scientists around the world presented in this book speaks volumes for the clinical potential of xeno factors such as resveratrol, quercetin, and others in terms of therapeutic gene activation. The outcome of ongoing clinical studies will hopefully confirm the value of these compounds.

Society and Living Longer

What if the pharmaceutical and nutraceutical companies that are now investing hundreds of millions of dollars in these life-extending compounds prove to be successful and actually do extend human life span? What are the implications of living just a few years longer, even if not to the 120-year mark projected by some scientists? Stanford University biologist Dr. Shripad Tuljapurkar concluded that between 2010 and 2030, antiaging therapies might be expected to increase the normal life span by twenty years. In more developed countries, the population of those sixty and over is expected to nearly double from 2005 to 2050. A research team headed by John R. Wilmoth studied life span in Sweden for the period between 1861 and 1999. These researchers concluded: "Our analysis refutes the common assertion that human life span is fixed and unchanging over time. . . . Reductions in death range ages, which have accelerated in recent decades, seem likely to continue, and may gradually extend the limits of achieved human longevity even further."

The downside of extending human life is that as people age, they consume more health-care resources. Some feel that the biggest threat to the United States over the next fifteen years comes not from terrorism or global warming but from a medical health system running amok. Those of us over sixty-five spend three times more for health care than the average younger person. Declining health after sixty-five results in major increases in the use of prescription drugs, hospital services, surgery, replacement of body parts, rehabilitation, physical therapy, and community-based services. The Employee Benefit Research Institute recently estimated that a sixty-five-year-old couple would need $440,000 of health-care funding if they lived until age ninety. They would need $778,000 to survive to the century mark. Those ninety and older already make up the fastest-growing segment of the U.S. population.

Quantity versus Quality

This raises a fundamental question: would an increase in life expectancy probably be accompanied by a prolonged deterioration in the quality of life? Or could we live longer, enjoying good health and increased satisfaction, by preventing or delaying the diseases that are now attendant on aging? These questions are the focus of policy planners in many organizations, including the International Union for the Scientific Study of Population. So important is this issue of quality of life that measures have been developed to take into account not only mortality or death but also the health status of the elderly. One index, called the Healthy Life Expectancy Index, was devised to measure life expectancy free of disease, or more particularly, the expectancy of living without limitations imposed by chronic disease.

Unsurprisingly, pessimists and optimists have lined up on opposite sides of this question of longevity versus quality of life. The pessimists say that by extending survival, we are encouraging a progressively more difficult battle against the disorders of old age. Tampering with the biological clock, they say, will just add years of suffering and put further strain on our already overcrowded nursing homes.

The optimists say that an increase in life expectancy can indeed be accompanied by maintaining quality of life. They point out that not all elderly persons experience deterioration in the quality of their lives. Some at seventy-five or eighty years of age have the functional ability of those decades younger. Support for this notion also comes from the New England Centenarian Study. As Dr. Thomas Perls reports, "Consistent with our hypothesis that centenarians markedly delay or even escape age-associated diseases—in other words, heart attack, stroke, cancer, diabetes and Alzheimer's—we noted that 90 percent of them were functionally independent for the vast majority of their lives up until the average age of ninety-two years, and 75 percent were the same at an average age of ninety-five years." Centenarians, therefore, disprove the perception that the older you get, the sicker you get. Centenarians teach us that the older you get, the healthier you've been.

I wrote earlier about Alzheimer's disease being the most common disorder causing dementia in the elderly, particularly after age sixty. Evidence is now accumulating, however, that agents such as omega-3 fatty acids found in fish and fish oil, physical and mental exercise, xeno factors, and other supplements all may reduce or delay the onset of this condition. History also substantiates that "use it or lose it" applies to our minds as well as our bodies. Michelangelo completed his final frescoes in the Vatican's Pauline Chapel at age seventy-five. Benjamin Franklin invented bifocal glasses at age seventy-eight to correct his own poor vision—even though it appears that he did not strictly adhere to his own adage "To live long, eat less"! Giuseppe Verdi finished his last opera, *Falstaff,* at age seventy-nine. Georgia O'Keeffe, despite failing vision, continued painting into her seventies. Frank Lloyd Wright nearly finished New York's Guggenheim Museum before his death at age ninety-one, and Martha Graham not only danced until age seventy-six but also choreographed for another twenty years.

The driving force behind the rapidly growing global phenomenon of antiaging is to maintain the quality of life. By providing a comprehensive preventive approach to medicine, rejuvenation and longevity— and even weight loss—become secondary by-products. Unfortunately, all too few physicians and health-care practitioners devote much time to preventive medicine. They are rewarded financially for fixing people's health after it breaks down, not for maintenance. Similarly, the profits of pharmaceutical companies are dependent on age-related diseases rather than on their prevention, with the exception of companies dedicated to decreasing or preventing the diseases of aging (see table 12).

The estimated cost per additional year of healthy life for drugs specifically targeting the diseases of aging is $8,790 per life year. This is roughly half the cost of stroke treatment, one-tenth the cost of cardiac defibrillators, and one-fifteenth the cost of diabetes prevention. This area of research may be the most effective in the area of preventive medicine.

Only through preventive medical maintenance will we be able to compress the dying process into the shortest possible time frame before we go gently into that good night. I do not believe that one pill or

TABLE 12 Cost-Benefit Analysis of Selected Future Therapies
(Adapted from Goldman et al., Rand study)

	Annual Treatment Cost ($ Billions)		Cost Per Additional Life Year ($)
	2015	2030	
Antiaging compound (healthy)	48.6	72.8	8,790
Cancer vaccines	0.5	0.8	18,236
Treatment of acute stroke	3.1	4.4	21,905
Telomerase inhibitors	4.4	6.4	61,884
Alzheimer's prevention	33.6	49.1	80,334
Intraventricular cardiodefibrillators	14.0	20.7	103,095
Diabetes prevention	13.7	20.96	147,199
Antiangiogenesis	38.8	51.9	496,809
Left ventricular assist devices	10.2	14.2	511,962
Pacemaker for atrial fibrillation	10.4	13.6	1,403,740

elixir will ever accomplish this completely, but it may play an important role. Throughout this book, we have seen how diet and an understanding of the new field of nutrigenomics can help to delay or prevent many of the diseases of aging.

In addition to good nutrition, the beneficial aspects of exercise—both physical and mental—have generated volumes of supportive research. We now know that physical exercise strengthens muscle and bone to reduce frailty and osteoporosis, and increases growth factors to enhance brain function, including memory. Challenging mental tasks, from card games to crossword puzzles to sudoku, increase brainpower in much the way that physical exercise strengthens muscles. Experiments show that the brains of laboratory animals grow larger when these animals are put in new mazes, and they live longer if stimulation is maintained. Stress of any kind, if chronic, causes deterioration of both the mind and the body. A strong faith associated with spirituality, meditation, and a supportive social setting all are essential in old age to mitigate the damaging effects of depression and the gradual diminishment of our physical powers.

From my reading and my experience dealing with thousands of patients, I come down firmly on the optimists' side of the debate over longevity versus quality of life. My personal goal is not to live 120 or 130 years but to maintain my present quality of life for as long as possible. To that end, I will continue to exercise my body and mind, cultivate family and friends, and extend altruism and kindness to my patients. Finally, I intend to continue to supplement my daily glass of Pinot Noir wine with natural xeno factors.

There are currently hundreds of dietary supplements for sale by various manufacturers that contain stressed plant polyphenols, including resveratrol. They have various concentrations and various degrees of purity that we would not attempt to list. The purpose of this book is primarily to make you aware of recent scientific breakthroughs, to explain why this information is important and why taking these plant polyphenols as a dietary supplement may be right for you. It is my sincere hope that you will use this information along with any and all other sources available to you to make an informed decision.

As we enter this new and exciting era of exploring the human genome and discovering previously hidden segments of our DNA code, we can think back to a time before modern drugs and chemicals when it was the food we ate that kept us healthy and strong. As a species, to stay alive from day to day we needed nutrients from plants, plants that have coevolved with animals and humans since the beginning of animal life on earth. Plants, and the amazing small molecules that they produce under stress, have provided humans an edge in our struggle for survival, and now they may offer us the key to achieving a more ambitious goal: living long and living well.

Appendix A:
Classification of Xeno Factors

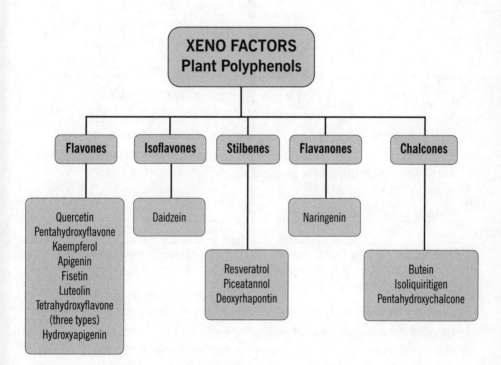

FIGURE 22 Classification of xeno factors/polyphenols.

Food Sources and Known Uses

STILBENES—RESVERATROL

Food Sources: Red-skin grapes, peanuts, tea, red wines, mulberries

Other Sources: Polygonum cuspidatum, eucalyptus, spruce, and lily

Known Uses: Antioxidant, anticancer, anti-inflammatory, decreases platelet aggregation, reduces LDL oxidation, phytoestrogen cardio-protectant properties, prolongs life in test animals, improves endurance and muscle strength, mitochondria neogenesis, inhibits weight gain, antifungal, antibacterial

TANNINS

Proanthocyanidins

Food Sources: Red grapes, all colors of berries, red wine, chocolate, cranberry, pomegranates, peaches, persimmons, apples, pears, cider, tea, beer, pine bark

Known Uses: Antioxidant, strengthens collagen, vasodilation, cardioprotective

Procyanidins

Food Sources: Chocolate, red wine, red grape seeds and skin

Known Uses: Antioxidant cardioprotective, lowers blood pressure

LIGNANS

Food Sources: Flaxseed (not flax oil), sesame seed, cereals (rye, wheat, oat, barley), pumpkin seeds, soybeans, broccoli, beans, and some berries

Known Uses: Acts as a phytoestrogen and cardioprotective, some cancer-risk reduction in women

OTHER POLYPHENOLS—CURCUMIN

Food Sources: Turmeric (yellow curry)

Known Uses: Anti-inflammatory, anticancer effects, found to reduce the progression of arthritis, heart disease, Alzheimer's disease, multiple sclerosis (MS), and depression

PHENOLIC ACIDS—REDUCE OXIDATION OF LDL, ANTICANCER EFFECTS

Ellagic Acid

Food Sources: Strawberries, raspberries

Known Uses: Reduces esophageal and colon cancers

Chlorogenic Acid

Food Sources: Blueberries, tomatoes, bell peppers, grapes, coffee

Known Uses: Antioxidant and anticancer, reduces oxidation of LDL

Cooking Facts: Roasting coffee beans increases antioxidant activity

Other Phenolic Acids (phytic acid, p-coumaric acid, ferulic acid, vanillin, cinnamic acid, hydroxycinnamic acids)

Food Sources: Red and green bell peppers, legumes, whole grains, wheat bran, brown rice, oats, apples, artichokes, peanuts, pineapple, potatoes, vanilla bean, cinnamon, blueberries, red and white grapes, flaxseed

Known Uses: Antioxidant for the colon mucosa, binds calcium and iron, reduces cancer and cardiovascular disease, antifungal, antiparasitic

for Xeno Factor/Polyphenols by Category

FLAVONOIDS—ANTIOXIDANTS AND ANTI-INFLAMMATORY

Flavanones

HESPERIDIN
Food Sources: Oranges, citrus fruits

Known Uses: Antioxidant, regenerates vitamin C, anticancer and antivirus effects

NARINGIN
Food Sources: Grapefruit

Known Uses: Reduces LDL cholesterol, reduces certain drug absorption, antioxidant activity, skin radiation protection

RUTIN
Food Sources: Asparagus, buckwheat, citrus fruits

Known Uses: Improves blood vessel wall strength

Flavonols

QUERCETIN AND KAEMPFEROL
(MOST COMMON FLAVONOIDS)

Food Sources: Apple skins, red onions, leeks, kale, buckwheat, red grapes, green tea

Known Uses: Antioxidant, cardiac benefits (reduces LDL, oxidation, vasodilator, and blood thinner), antivirus, reduction of allergic response

MYRICETIN
Food Sources: Cherry tomato, broccoli, blueberry, black currant, apricot, beans, red wine

Known Uses: Antioxidant, cardiac benefits (reduces LDL, oxidation, vasodilator, and blood thinner), antivirus, reduction of allergic response

Flavones

APIGENIN AND LUTEOLIN
Food Sources: Parsley, celery, millet, wheat, skin of citrus fruit

Known Uses: Antioxidant, may protect against autoimmune diseases such as MS

Flavonols

CATECHINS (EPIGALLOCATECHIN GALLEATE [EGCG], EPICATECHIN, EPIGALLOCATECHIN)

Food Sources: Dark (70 percent cacao) chocolate, tea (green/white), cranberries, apricots, beans, cherry, red grapes, peach, blackberry, apple, red wine, cider

Known Uses: Reduces cancer, inhibits proinflammatory factors (NF-κB) associated with cancer and inflammation

Anthocyanins (color pigments)

CYANIDIN—MOST COMMON

Food Sources: Red wine, cherries, strawberries, blueberries, red grapes, blackberries, black raspberries, cereals, cabbage, onion, beans, radishes

Known Uses: Protects cells from oxidative damage

Cooking Facts: Heat (cooking) removes this nutrient.

Isoflavones—similar to estrogen Genistein, glycitein, and daidzein

Food Sources: Soybeans, tofu, soy milk, legumes, pomegranate seeds

Known Uses: elevates HDL cholesterol and lowers LDL cholesterol, antioxidants and has a phytoestrogen effect to reduce cardiovascular risk and smooth menopause symptoms and onset of osteoporosis in women; has anticancer effects.

Appendix B: Timeline of Discovery

Year	Scientist(s)	Discovery
1859	Charles Darwin	Published *On the Origin of Species* and the theory of natural selection
1866	Gregor Mendel	Published "Experiments in Plant Hybridization" and demonstrates the laws of inheritance
1902	Walter Sutton	Demonstrated that chromosomes exist in similar pairs within the nucleus of cells
1909	Wilhelm Johannsen	Danish botanist who coined the word *gene* (origin or to give birth) to describe the functional units of heredity
1927	Hermann Joseph Muller	Used X-ray to cause artificial gene mutations in the fruit fly *Drosophila*
1935	Clive McCay	Discovered that calorie restriction without malnutrition prolongs lives of rats
1941	George W. Beadle and Edward L. Tatum	Discovered that genes control the production of enzymes, biochemical catalysts made of proteins
1943	Erwin Schrödinger	Stated that DNA was paired in the cell nucleus and contained the "code of life"
1944	Oswald T. Avery	Purified DNA and stated that it was responsible for heredity

1951	Erwin Chargaff	Observed that base pairs in DNA were "coupled" adenine-thymine, guanine-cytosine
1951	Rosalind Franklin	First obtained sharp X-ray diffraction pictures of DNA
1953	James Watson and Francis Crick	Building on the work of Rosalind Franklin, published the structure of DNA and the double helix containing the code of life
1956	Denham Harman	Published free-radical theory of aging
1961	Leonard Hayflick	Documented that the replicative life span of a normal human cell—the number of times it can reproduce itself—is limited (the "Hayflick limit")
1974	Sydney Brenner	Developed the roundworm *C. elegans* as a laboratory model to study genetic manipulations
1983	Michael Klass	Demonstrated that mutant strains of roundworms could be isolated and longevity dramatically altered
1988	D. B. Friedman and Thomas Johnson	Building on the work of Michael Klass, demonstrated for the first time that the mutation of a single gene, age-1, can extend life in the worm
1993	Cynthia Kenyon	Discovered genetic links between longevity and insulin signaling and more than doubled the life span of roundworms
1994	Gordon Lithgow and Tom Johnson	Discovered genetic mutations that extend a worm's life also make the worms more resistant to stress, supporting the concept that increasing a cell's resistance to stress delays aging
1995	Brian Kennedy and Leonard Guarente	Discovered that manipulation of silencing proteins in yeast cells can substantially increase their life span

(continued)

Year	Scientist(s)	Discovery
1996	Holly Brown-Borg and Andrej Bartke	Reported the discovery that a single-gene mutation can influence longevity in a mammal, acting through a pathway similar to the one shown by Cynthia Kenyon in worms
1997	David Sinclair and Leonard Guarente	Discovered a genetic explanation for yeast cell aging, making yeast the only organism for which the cause of aging is known
1998	Andrea Bodnar, Michelle Oullette, Jerry Shay, Woody Wright	Demonstrated that telomerase, an enzyme that stabilizes telomere length, removes the Hayflick limit, allowing human cells to divide indefinitely
1999	Matt Kaeberlein and Leonard Guarente	Showed that the Silent Information Regulator 2 (SIR2) gene controls longevity in yeast cells
2000	Su-Ju Lin and Leonard Guarente	Discovered link among sirtuin gene activation, caloric restriction, and aging in yeast
2001	Francis Collins and Craig Venter	Announced the sequencing of a rough draft of the human genome
2001	Heidi Tissenbaum and Leonard Guarente	Showed that the SIR2 gene can extend life span in worms and suggested that it also modulates the healthful effects of calorie restriction on other organisms
2003	Konrad Howitz and David Sinclair	Provided first evidence that resveratrol activates SIR2 (the protein encoded by the SIR2 gene) and extends the life span of yeast; also described the xenohormesis hypothesis
2004	Blanka Rogina and Stephen Helfand	Showed that SIR2 controls life span in flies and is required for life-span extension by caloric restriction
2004	Jason Wood and David Sinclair	Demonstrated that resveratrol extends the life spans of worms and flies

2006	Dario Valenzano and Alessandro Cellerino	Showed that resveratrol extends life span in a vertebrate fish
2006	Joseph Baur, Kevin Pearson, Rafael de Cabo, David Sinclair	Discovered multiple health and longevity benefits of resveratrol in obese mice
2006	Marie Lagouge, Carmen Argmann, Johan Auwerx	Discovered weight-suppressing effects of resveratrol, along with increased mitochondrial production and increased endurance
2008	David Sinclair and Rafael de Cabo	Demonstrated that resveratrol delays age-related deterioration and mimics genetic changes similar to those of dietary restriction but without extending life span
2008	Konrad Howitz and David Sinclair	Showed that xenohormesis activation is the result of other species' sensing the chemical and environmental cues
2008	Tomas Prolla and Richard Weindruch	Demonstrated that low doses of resveratrol can mimic caloric restriction effects and retard aging in mice

Appendix C: Existing Patents and NIH-Funded Clinical Trials

Existing Patents and Resveratrol

Pharmascience, a Montreal-based pharmaceutical company, was awarded a patent for the use of trans-resveratrol to prevent and to treat restenosis after coronary disease treatment.

The Institute of Human Virology, funded by Pharmascience, has filed a patent application for the use of resveratrol with nucleoside analogs for treating HIV-1 infections.

Trans-resveratrol
[501-36-0]

Review of Toxicological Literature, *Prepared for* Scott Masten, PhD
National Institute of Environmental Health Sciences
P.O. Box 12233
Research Triangle Park, NC 27709
Contract No. N01-ES-65402

Submitted by
Karen E. Haneke, M.S.
Integrated Laboratory Systems
P.O. Box 13501
Research Triangle Park, NC 27709
March 2002

Commercial Availability

Several companies produce *trans*-resveratrol commercially. Pharmascience of Montreal, Canada, produces a pure form of *trans*-resveratrol (PCT Gazette, 2001; Agriculture and Agri-Food Canada, undated). InterHealth of Concord, CA (InterHealth, undated-a), produces a standardized extract of *trans*-resveratrol. Pharmascience calls its patented product Resverin® (PCT Gazette, 2001; Pharmascience, undated; Agriculture and Agri-Food Canada, undated; Food and Beverage America, 2000). InterHealth manufactures Protykin™, a standardized extract containing *trans*-resveratrol and emodin, also a polyphenol, from the dried rhizome of *P. cuspidatum* (InterHealth, undated-a,b,c,d). Laboratorio Italiano Biochimico Farmaceutical Lisapharma has patented a pharmaceutical composition of grape and wine polyphenols, particularly resveratrol, with yeast (Osterwalder, 1999). Other manufacturers of *trans*-resveratrol include TCI America of Portland, OR; LKT Laboratories of St. Paul, MN; and Samlong Chemical Co., Ltd., of China (Block, 2000; LKT Laboratories, Inc., undated; Samlong Chemical Co., Ltd., undated; TCI America, 1999). Moravek Biochemicals of Brea, CA, produces radiolabeled resveratrol (Moravek Biochemicals, 2001)

Pharmascience has a patent for use of *trans*-resveratrol to prevent and to treat restenosis after coronary disease treatment (AML Information Services, 2000), and the Institute for Human Virology, funded by Pharmascience, has filed a patent application for the use of resveratrol with nucleoside analogs for treating HIV-1 infections (IHV, 2001a,b).

Agriculture and Agri-Food Canada. Undated. Functional foods and nutraceuticals: Pharmascience, Inc. Internet address: http://www.agr.ca/food/markets/nutraceu/Profiles2000E/phrmasci.html. Last accessed on April 9, 2001.

Pharmascience. Undated. Resverin®. Internet address://www.pharmascience.com-/pms_en/health/3_1_6.ASP. Last accessed on July 18, 2001.

Pharmascience. Undated. Partnerships and Alliances. Internet address: http://www.Pharmascience.com/pms_en/about/1_1_6.asp. Last accessed on July 18, 2001.

Clinical Studies on Resveratrol

1. Resveratrol for Patients with Colon Cancer
    Condition: Colon Cancer

Purpose

Resveratrol has been found to modulate Wnt signaling, a signaling pathway that is activated in over 85 percent of colon cancers. In this proposal, studies will be performed to define the actions of resveratrol on the Wnt signaling pathway in a clinical trial in which patients with colon cancer who will receive treatment with resveratrol and correlative laboratory studies will examine its effects directly on colon cancer and normal colonic mucosa. These studies will provide data on the mechanisms of resveratrol action and provide a foundation for future prevention trials, correlative studies, and therapeutic clinical research with this agent.

2. Resveratrol in Preventing Cancer in Healthy Participants
    Condition: Unspecified Adult Solid Tumor, Protocol Specific

Purpose

Chemoprevention is the use of certain drugs to keep cancer from forming, growing, or coming back. The use of resveratrol may prevent cancer. This phase I trial is studying the side effects and best dose of resveratrol in preventing cancer in healthy participants.

3. Resveratrol in Treating Patients with Colorectal Cancer That Can Be Removed By Surgery
    Condition: Colorectal Cancer

Purpose

Resveratrol may stop the growth of tumor cells by blocking some of the enzymes needed for cell growth. This phase I trial is studying the side effects and best dose of resveratrol in treating patients with colorectal cancer that can be removed by surgery.

4. Dietary Intervention in Follicular Lymphoma
    Condition: Follicular Lymphoma

Purpose

A dietary intervention study in patients with stage III/IV follicular lymphoma (FL) to assess the ability of several dietary factors to induce cell death, inhibit cell proliferation, and control how tumor cells infiltrate normal tissue.

Appendix D: Partial List of Fish Oil Supplements and Multivitamins

Nordic Naturals Omega-3 Purified Fish Oil (165 milligrams EPA and 110 milligrams DHA per soft gel, 2 per day)

Manufactured by Nordic Naturals

GNC Fish Body Oils (180 milligrams EPA and 120 milligrams DHA per soft gel, 3–6 per day)

Distributed by General Nutrition Corporation

OmegaGuard™—pharmaceutical grade fish oil (545 milligrams EPA and 360 milligrams DHA per 3 softgels)

Distributed by Shaklee Corporation

Omega/Rx (400 milligrams EPA and 200 milligrams DHA per soft gel, 4 per day)

Manufactured by Zone Labs

Jarrow Formulas Max DHA 600 milligrams Omega-3 per gram, 420 DHA per gram (36 milligrams EPA and 250 milligrams DHA per soft gel, 1–6 per day)

Distributed by Jarrow Formulas

Weil—Andrew Weil, MD, Omega-3 Complex (333 milligrams EPA and 167 milligrams DHA per soft gel, 1 per day)

Manufactured by IdeaSphere

Mega Men Multivitamin

Distributed by General Nutrition Corporation

Life Extension Mix Caps

Distributed by Life Extension Foundation

Acknowledgments

This is an opportunity for me to make amends for the fact that this book should have been published with two additional authors: David Sinclair and Jeffrey Bost. As director of the Paul F. Glenn Laboratories for the Biological Mechanisms of Aging at Harvard University, Dr. Sinclair is responsible for research into the genetic mechanisms of aging, which provides the underpinnings for the revolutionary theory that stressed plants, particularly grapes, "talk" to people in ways that increase longevity, memory, and overall health. For this, and for the many hours he spent with me explaining the molecular biology of aging, from yeast to man, I express my deepest gratitude.

Jeff Bost, PAC, a colleague and friend for twenty-one years, has also provided invaluable research for these pages, which includes his designing, along with James Smoliga, PhD, the first human clinical research protocol to assess resveratrol, quercetin, and the Australian extract. Without Jeff's tireless efforts, encouragement, and skills, this book would not have happened.

I am also deeply indebted to Joe Baur, David Sinclair's colleague at the Paul F. Glenn Laboratories for the Biological Mechanisms of Aging at Harvard University and a longevity pioneer in his own right. Joe dissected the manuscript of this book for accuracy and graciously provided the foreword, for which I am indebted to him. Peter Guzzardi, editor for Stephen Hawking, Deepak Chopra, and Queen Noor, applied his consummate editing skills to separate the wheat from the chaff—at times painfully, but always to good effect. And copy editor Philip Bashe was remarkably thorough and attentive to detail.

Sanjay Gupta, a neurosurgeon, and Mehmet Oz, a cardiac surgeon, were inspirational in the writing of this book. Although surgery is an art form, it is also piecework: treating one patient's disease at a time. But how much better it is to broadly prevent illness before it arises than fight to correct it once it has taken hold. Besides being masters themselves in the arts of brain and heart surgery, both of these surgeons have committed themselves to *preventing* many of the diseases they treat surgically. Through their books and other media, they reach millions of people with the all-important message that a healthy lifestyle, proper nutrition, and a balanced life are the cornerstones of preventive medicine. In this book I have attempted to follow their example and expand upon their all-important messages.

My friend Greg Norman provided encouragement and critical support by introducing me to Judith Curr and Peter Borland at Atria Books. They took a leap of faith by agreeing to publish this book after seeing a two-page proposal, and have been wonderfully supportive—and patient—throughout.

Peter and Lynda Voigt graciously showed me firsthand Peter's ingenious extraction process, welcoming me to their home on the Mornington Peninsula in Australia and adding immensely to the "Australian Extract" section.

For more than a decade, Dennis and Rose Heindl and the Mylan Laboratories Charitable Foundation, under the direction of founder Milan Puskar and Robert Coury, CEO, have provided financial support to my laboratory and to my academic career at the University of Pittsburgh, for which I will be forever grateful.

For twenty years as team neurosurgeon for the Pittsburgh Steelers I have witnessed firsthand the importance of endurance, strength, and reaction time in professional athletes. I wish to thank Mr. Dan Rooney and Mr. Art Rooney for giving me this extraordinary opportunity.

Many scientists, colleagues, friends, and family members gave tirelessly of their time to review and discuss the manuscript. My heartfelt thanks to my dearest friend, Margaret Scherbel, and to Paula and David Sculley, Bill Watts, Mark Juliano, Bryan Donahue, and my extended family, Laura, Lisa, Adara, Isabella, Jonathan, Mary, Lorraine, Cynthia, and Lynn. I also deeply thank Karen Hlavac for the many hours she patiently spent transcribing and editing my thousands of notes, and Jon Coulter for his compelling artwork and illustrations. Also included among the scientists are David Sinclair's coinvestigators and pioneers in aging in their own right: Johan Auwerx, discoverer of the endurance phenotype; Konrad Howitz, codiscoverer of resveratrol's ability to activate SIRT1; Rafael de Cabo and Kevin Pearson, main collaborators on the life-span extension experiment that garnered international acclaim; Cynthia Kenyon; and Leonard Guarente.

To all of you, and to the many more who have helped me in countless ways as I worked on this book, I extend my deepest appreciation.

References

CHAPTER 1: THE ORIGINS OF LIFE

1. J. D. Watson and F. H. Crick, "The structure of DNA," *Cold Spring Harbor Symposia on Quantum Biology* 18 (1953): 123–131.
2. K. T. Howitz, K. J. Bitterman, H. Y. Cohen, D. W. Lamming, et al., "Small molecule activators of sirtuins extend Saccharomyces cerevisiae lifespan," *Nature* 425 (6954) (September 11, 2003): 191–196.
3. D. W. Lamming, J. G. Wood, and D. A. Sinclair, "Small molecules that regulate lifespan: evidence for xenohormesis," *Molecular Microbiology* 53 (4) (August 2004): 1003–1009.
4. K. T. Howitz and D. Sinclair, "Xenohormesis: sensing the chemical cues of other species," *Cell* 133 (3) (May 2, 2008): 387–391.
5. L. Bordone and L. Guarente, "Calorie restriction, SIRT1 and metabolism: understanding longevity," *Nature Reviews Molecular and Cell Biology* 6 (April 2005): 298–305.
6. S. J. Lin, P. A. Defossez, and L. Guarente, "Requirement of NAD and SIR2 for life-span extension by calorie restriction in Saccharomyces cerevisiae," *Science* 289 (September 22, 2000): 2126–2128.
7. N. Arantes-Oliveira, J. Apfeld, A. Dillin, and C. Kenyon, "Regulation of life-span by germ-line stem cells in Caenorhabditis elegans," *Science* 295 (5554) (January 18, 2002): 502–505.
8. A. Dillin, D. K. Crawford, and C. Kenyon, "Timing requirements for insulin/IGF-1 signaling in C. elegans," *Science* 298 (5594) (October 25, 2002): 830–834.
9. J. Apfeld and C. Kenyon, "Cell nonautonomy of C. elegans daf-2 function in the regulation of diapause and life span," *Cell* 95 (2) (October 16, 1998): 199–210.
10. H. Hsin and C. Kenyon, "Signals from the reproductive system regulate the lifespan of C. elegans," *Nature* 399 (6734) (May 27, 1999): 362–366.
11. K. Lin, H. Hsin, N. Libina, and C. Kenyon, "Regulation of the Caenorhabditis elegans longevity protein DAF-16 by insulin/IGF-1 and germline signaling," *Nature Genetics* 28 (2) (June 2001): 139–145.

12. A. Dillin, D. K. Crawford, and C. Kenyon, "Timing requirements for insulin/IGF-1 signaling in C. elegans," *Science* 298 (5594) (October 25, 2002): 830–834.
13. Steven Weinberg, *The first three minutes: a modern view of the origin of the universe* (New York: Basic Books, 1993).

CHAPTER 2: MOLECULAR PIONEERS AND THE DISCOVERY OF LONGEVITY GENES

1. J. D. Watson and F. H. Crick, "Molecular structure of nucleic acids; a structure for deoxyribose nucleic acid," *Nature* 171 (4356) (April 25, 1953): 737–738.
2. Charles Darwin, *On the origin of species by means of natural selection, or the preservation of favoured races in the struggle for life* (London: John Murray, 1859).
3. C. Wilson and J. W. Szostak, "Ribozyme catalysis," *Current Opinion in Structural Biology* 2 (5) (October 1992): 749–756.
4. Carl Woese, *The genetic code* (New York: Harper & Row, 1968).
5. Carl Sagan, *The dragons of Eden: speculations on the evolution of human intelligence* (New York: Random House, 1977).
6. R. A. Fisher, "Has Mendel's work been rediscovered?" *Annals of Science* 1 (1936): 115–137.
7. Michel Morange, *A history of molecular biology* (Cambridge, MA: Harvard University Press, 1998).

CHAPTER 3: CAUSES OF AGING

1. L. Hayflick, "Biological aging is no longer an unsolved problem," *Annals of the New York Academy of Sciences* 1100 (April 2007): 1–13.
2. L. A. Talbot, C. H. Morrell, J. L. Fleg, and E. J. Metter, "Changes in leisure time physical activity and risk of all-cause mortality in men and women: the Baltimore longitudinal study of aging," *Preventive Medicine* 45 (2–3) (August–September 2007): 169–176.
3. *Posing questions/finding answers,* National Institute on Aging, free publications online, www.niapublications.org/pubs/microscope/chapter1.pdf.
4. J. P. de Magalhães, C. E. Finch, J. M. Sedivy, S. N. Austad, et al., "A proposal to sequence genomes of unique interest for research on aging," *Journals of Gerontology Series A: Biological Sciences and Medical Sciences* 62 (6) (June 2007): 583–584.
5. L. A. Gavrilov and N. S. Gavrilova, "The reliability theory of aging and longevity," *Journal of Theoretical Biology* 213 (4) (December 21, 2001): 527–545.

6. Peter Brian Medawar, *An unsolved problem of biology* (London: H. K. Lewis, 1952).
7. G. C. Williams, "Pleiotropy, natural selection and the evolution of senescence," *Evolution* 11 (4) (December 1957): 398–411.
8. T. Kirkwood and F. R. S. Holliday, "The evolution of ageing and longevity," *Proceedings of the Royal Society of London, Series B* 205 (1161) (September 21, 1979): 531–546.
9. Theodore C. Goldsmith, *The evolution of aging,* 2nd ed. (Crownsville, MD: Azinet Press, 2006).
10. T. C. Goldsmith, "Aging, evolvability, and the individual benefit requirement: medical implications of theory controversies," *Journal of Theoretical Biology* 252 (4) (June 21, 2008): 764–768.
11. J. Mitteldorf, "Chaotic population dynamics and the evolution of ageing," *Evolutionary Ecology Research* 8 (2006): 561–574.
12. T. C. Goldsmith, "Aging as an evolved characteristic—Weismann's theory reconsidered," *Medical Hypotheses* 62 (2) (February 2004): 304–308.
13. R. Weindruch, R. L. Walford, S. Fligiel, and D. Guthrie, "The retardation of aging in mice by dietary restriction: longevity, cancer, immunity and lifetime energy intake," *Journal of Nutrition* 116 (4) (April 1986): 641–654.
14. M. A. Lane, D. K. Ingram, and G. S. Roth, "The serious search for an anti-aging pill," *Scientific American* 287 (2) (August 2002): 36–41.
15. N. Arantes-Oliveira, J. Apfeld, A. Dillin, and C. Kenyon, "Regulation of life-span by germ-line stem cells in Caenorhabditis elegans," *Science* 295 (5554) (January 18, 2002): 502–505.
16. H. S. Lodge, "You can stop 'normal' aging," *Parade,* March 18, 2007.
17. D. Rudman, A. G. Feller, H. S. Nagraj, G. A. Gergans, et al., "Effects of human growth hormone in men over 60 years old," *New England Journal of Medicine* 323 (1) (July 5, 1990): 1–6.
18. M. R. Blackman, J. D. Sorkin, T. Münzer, M. F. Bellantoni, et al., "Growth hormone and sex steroid administration in healthy aged women and men: a randomized controlled trial," *Journal of the American Medical Association* 288 (18) (November 13, 2002): 2282–2292.
19. M. A. Papadakis, D. Grady, D. Black, M. Tierney, et al., "Growth hormone replacement in older men improves body composition but not functional ability," *Annals of Internal Medicine* 124 (8) (April 15, 1996): 708–716.
20. D. R. Taaffe, L. Pruitt, J. Reim, R. L. Hintz, et al., "Effect of recombinant human growth hormone on the muscle strength response to resistance exercise in elderly men," *Journal of Clinical Endocrinology and Metabolism* 79 (5) (November 1994): 1361–1366.
21. M. L. Vance, "Can growth hormone prevent aging?," *New England Journal of Medicine,* 348 (9) (February 27, 2003): 779–780.

22. M. L. Vance, "Growth hormone for the elderly?," *New England Journal of Medicine* 323 (1) (July 5, 1990): 52–54.
23. N.-W. Kim, M. A. Piatyszek, K. R. Prowse, C. B. Harley, et al., "Specific association of human telomerase activity with immortal cells and cancer," *Science* 266 (5193) (December 23, 1994): 2011–2015.
24. S. L. Weinrich, R. Pruzan, L. Ma, M. Ouelette, et al., "Reconstitution of telomerase with the catalytic protein subunit hTERT," *Nature Genetics* 17 (4) (December 1997): 498–502.
25. A. G. Bodnar, M. Ouellete, M. Frolkis, S. E. Holt, et al., "Extension of life span by introduction of telomerase in normal human cells," *Science* 279 (5349) (January 16, 1998): 349–352.
26. J. W. Shay, "Telomerase in cancer: Diagnostic, prognostic and therapeutic implications," *Cancer Journal from Scientific American* (4, supplement 1) (May 1998): S26–S34.
27. J. W. Shay and W. E. Wright, "The use of telomerized cells for tissue engineering," *Nature Biotechnology* 18 (1) (January 2000): 22–23.
28. *Aging under the microscope: a biological quest,* National Institute on Aging, NIH publication No. 02-2756.

CHAPTER 4: CALORIE RESTRICTION AND LONGEVITY

1. C. M. McCay, Mary F. Crowell, and L. A. Maynard, "The effect of retarded growth upon the length of life span and upon the ultimate body size," *Journal of Nutrition* 10 (1) (July 1935): 63–79.
2. C. M. McCay, L. A. Maynard, G. Sperling, and L. L. Barnes, "Retarded growth, life span, ultimate body size and age changes in the albino rat after feeding diets restricted in calories," *Journal of Nutrition* 18 (1) (July 1939): 1–13.
3. C. M. McCay and Mary F. Crowell, "Prolonging the lifespan," *Scientific Monthly* 39 (1934): 405–414.
4. Jeanette B. McCay, *Clive McCay: nutrition pioneer: biographical memoirs by his wife* (Mineral, VA: Tabby House Publishing, 1994).
5. E. M. Widdowson, "Physiological processes of aging: are there special nutritional requirements for elderly people? Do McCay's findings apply to humans?" *American Journal of Clinical Nutrition* 55 (6 supplement) (June 1992): 1246S–1249S.
6. Paul McGlothin and Meredith Averill, *The CR way* (New York: HarperCollins Publishers, 2008).
7. A. Keys, J. Brozek, A. Henschel, O. Mickelsen, et al., *The biology of human starvation* (Minneapolis: University of Minneapolis Press, 1950).
8. R. Weindruch and R. L. Walford, "Dietary restriction in mice beginning at 1 year of age: effect on life-span and spontaneous cancer incidence," *Science* 215 (4538) (March 12, 1982): 1415–1418.

9. M. P. Mattson, R. M. Anson, Z. Guo, R. de Cabo, et al., "Intermittent fasting dissociates beneficial effects of dietary restriction on glucose metabolism and neuronal resistance to injury from calorie intake," *Proceedings of the National Academy of Sciences of the United States of America* 100 (10) (May 13, 2003): 6216–6220.

10. E. J. Masoro, B. P. Yu, and H. A. Bertrand, "Action of food restriction in delaying the aging process," *Proceedings of the National Academy of Sciences of the United States of America* 79 (13) (July 1982): 4239–4241.

11. M. H. Ross, "Length of life and caloric intake," *American Journal of Clinical Nutrition* 25 (8) (August 1972): 834–838.

12. N. L. Bodkin, T. M. Alexander, H. K. Ortmeyer, E. Johnson, et al., "Mortality and morbidity in laboratory-maintained rhesus monkeys and effects of long-term dietary restriction," *Journals of Gerontology, Series A, Biological Sciences and Medical Sciences* 58 (3) (March 2003): 212–219.

13. L. M. Kalm and R. D. Semba, "They starved so that others be better fed: remembering Ancel Keys and the Minnesota experiment," *Journal of Nutrition* 135 (6) (June 2005): 1347–1352.

14. E. E. Calle, M. J. Thun, J. M. Petrelli, C. Rodriguez, et al., "Body-mass index and mortality in a prospective cohort of U.S. adults," *New England Journal of Medicine* 341 (15) (October 7, 1999): 1097–1105.

15. P. Cicconetti, L. Tafaro, G. Tedeschi, M. T. Tomolillo, et al., "Lifestyle and cardiovascular aging in centenarians," *Archives of Gerontology and Geriatrics* 35 (supplement) (2002): 93–98.

16. Brian M. Delaney and Lisa Walford, *The longevity diet: discover calorie restriction—the only proven way to slow the aging process and maintain peak vitality* (New York: Marlowe & Company, 2005).

17. L. Fontana and S. Klein, "Aging, adiposity, and calorie restriction," *Journal of the American Medical Association* 297 (9) (March 7, 2007): 986–994.

18. B. J. Willcox, K. Yano, R. Chen, D. C. Willcox, et al., "How much should we eat? The association between energy intake and mortality in a 36-year follow-up study of Japanese-American men," *Journals of Gerontology, Series A, Biological Sciences and Medical Sciences* 59 (8) (August 2004): 789–795.

19. D. T. Villareal, L. Fontana, E. P. Weiss, S. B. Racette, et al., "Bone mineral density response to caloric restriction–induced weight loss or exercise-induced weight loss: a randomized controlled trial," *Archives of Internal Medicine* 166 (22) (December 11–25, 2006): 2502–2510.

20. Roy L. Walford, *Beyond the 120-year diet* (New York: Four Walls Eight Windows, 2000).

21. H. Todoriki, D. C. Willcox, and B. J. Willcox. "The effects of post-war dietary change on longevity and health in Okinawa," *Okinawa Journal of American Studies* 1 (2004): 55–64.

22. L. K. Heilbronn, L. de Jonge, M. I. Frisard, J. P. DeLany, et al., "Effect of 6-month calorie restriction on biomarkers of longevity, metabolic adaptation, and oxidative stress in overweight individuals: a randomized controlled trial, *Journal of the American Medical Association* 295 (13) (April 5, 2006): 1539–1548.

23. T. E. Meyer, S. J. Kovács, A. A. Ehsani, S. Klein, et al., "Caloric restriction ameliorates the decline in diastolic function in humans," *Journal of the American College of Cardiology* 47 (2) (January 17, 2006): 398–402.

24. L. Sjöström, K. Narbro, C. D. Sjöström, K. Karason, et al. "Effects of bariatric surgery on mortality in Swedish obese subjects," *New England Journal of Medicine* 357 (8) (August 23, 2007): 741–752.

25. T. D. Adams, R. E. Gress, S. C. Smith, R. C. Halverson, et al., "Long-term mortality after gastric bypass surgery," *New England Journal of Medicine* 357 (8) (August 23, 2007): 753–761.

26. G. A. Bray, "The Missing Link—Lose Weight, Live Longer," *New England Journal of Medicine* 357 (8) (August 23, 2007): 818–820.

27. D. Harman, "Aging: a theory based on free radical and radiation chemistry." *Journal of Gerontology* 11 (3) (July 1956): 298–300.

28. D. Harman, "Free radical theory of aging: effect of free radical reaction inhibitors on the mortality rate of male LAF mice," *Journal of Gerontology* 23 (4) (October 1968): 476–482.

29. D. Harman, "The aging process: major risk factor for disease and death," *Proceedings of the National Academy of Sciences of the United States of America* 88 (12) (June 15, 1991): 5360–5363.

30. D. A. Sinclair and L. Guarente, "Unlocking the secrets of longevity genes," *Scientific American* 294 (3) (March 2006): 48–51, 54–57.

31. Sydney Brenner: The Nobel Prize in Physiology or Medicine 2002, Nobelprize.org, www.nobelprize.org/nobel_prizes/medicine/laureates/2002/brenner-autobio.html.

CHAPTER 5: BEGINNING TO UNDERSTAND LONGEVITY GENES

1. Sydney Brenner, *A life in science* (London: BioMed Central, 2001).

2. T. A. Abrams, D. J. Boocock, D. E. Brenner, G. E. S. Faust, et al., "Pilot study phase I single-dose safety and pharmacokinetics clinical study of resveratrol," protocol version 3.1 (December 16, 2004).

3. D. J. Boocock, D. E. Brenner, A. J. Gescher, W. P. Steward, et al., "Phase I repeat-dose clinical study of safety, pharmacokinetics and pharmacodynamics of resveratrol," NCI Division of Cancer Prevention, N01-CN-25025, protocol version 32.

4. J. Apfeld and C. Kenyon, "Cell nonautonomy of *C. elegans daf-2* function in the regulation of diapause and life span," *Cell* 95 (2) (October 16, 1998): 199–210.

5. D. B. Friedman and T. E. Johnson, "A mutation in the age-1 gene in *Caenorhabditis elegans* lengthens life and reduces hermaphrodite fertility genetics," *Genetics* 118 (1) (January 1988): 75–86.

6. M. R. Klass, "Aging in the nematode *Caenorhabditis elegans:* major biological and environmental factors influencing lifespan," *Mechanisms of Ageing and Development* 6 (6) (November–December 1977): 413–429.

7. M. R. Klass, "A method for the isolation of longevity mutants in the nematode *Caenorhabditis elegans* and initial results," *Mechanisms of Ageing and Development* 22 (3–4) (July–August 1983): 279–286.

8. M. R. Klass and D. Hirsh, "Nonageing developmental variant of *Caenorhabditis elegans,*" *Nature* 260 (5551) (April 8, 1976): 523–525.

9. Lenny Guarente, *Ageless quest: one scientist's search for genes that prolong youth* (Cold Spring Harbor, NY: Cold Spring Harbor Laboratory Press, 2003).

10. D. A. Sinclair and L. Guarente, "Extrachromosomal rDNA circles—a cause of aging in yeast," *Cell* 91 (7) (December 26, 1997): 1033–1042.

11. D. Esposito, G. Fassina, P. Szabo, P. De Angelis, et al., "Chromosomes of older humans are more prone to aminopterine-induced breakage," *Proceedings of the National Academy of Sciences of the United States of America* 86 (4) (February 1989): 1302–1306.

12. L. Guarente, "Mutant mice live longer," *Nature* 402 (6759) (November 18, 1999): 243–244.

13. R. M. Anderson, K. J. Bitterman, J. G. Wood, O. Medvedik, et al., "Nicotinamide and PNC1 govern lifespan extension by calorie restriction in *Saccharomyces cerevisiae,*" *Nature* 423 (6936) (May 8, 2003): 181–185.

14. R. M. Anderson, K. J. Bitterman, J. G. Wood, O. Medvedik, et al., "Manipulation of a nuclear NAD+ salvage pathway delays aging without altering steady-state NAD+ levels," *Journal of Biological Chemistry* 277 (21) (May 24, 2002): 18881–18890.

15. K. T. Howitz and D. Sinclair, "Xenohormesis: sensing the chemical cues of other species," *Cell* 133 (3) (May 2, 2008): 387–391.

16. K. T. Howitz, K. J. Bitterman, H.Y. Cohen, D. W. Lamming, et al., "Small molecule activators of sirtuins extend *Saccharomyces cerevisiae* lifespan," *Nature* 425 (6954) (September 11, 2003): 191–196.

17. H. Yang, J. A. Baur, A. Chen, C. Miller, et al., "Design and synthesis of compounds that extend yeast replicative lifespan," *Aging Cell* 6 (1) (February 2007): 35–43.

18. J. Baur and D. Sinclair, "Therapeutic potential of resveratrol: the in vivo evidence," *Nature Reviews Drug Discovery* 5 (June 2006): 493–505.

19. J. A. Baur, K. J. Pearson, N. L. Price, H. A. Jamieson, et al., "Resveratrol improves health and survival of mice on a high-calorie diet," *Nature* 444 (November 16, 2006): 337–342.

20. Konrad T. Howitz and David A. Sinclair, "Xenohormesis: sensing the chemical cues of other species," *Cell* 133 (3) (May 2, 2008): 387–391.

21. Kevin J. Pearson, David A. Sinclair, and Rafael de Cabo, "Resveratrol delays age-related deterioration and mimics transcriptional aspects of dietary restriction without extending life span," *Cell Metabolism* 8 (2) (August 2008): 157–168.

CHAPTER 6: THE FRENCH PARADOX
AND THE HOLY GRAIL OF AGING

1. R. Corder, W. Mullen, N. Q. Khan, S. C. Marks, et al., "Oenology: red wine procyanidins and vascular health," *Nature* 444 (7119) (November 30, 2006): 566.

2. D. R. Valenzano, E. Terzibasi, T. Genade, A. Cattaneo, et al., "Resveratrol prolongs lifespan and retards the onset of age-related markers in a short-lived vertebrate," *Current Biology* 16 (3) (February 7, 2006): 296–300.

3. J. Baur, K. J. Pearson, N. L. Price, H. A. Jamieson, et al., "Resveratrol improves health and survival of mice on a high-calorie diet," *Nature* 444 (7117) (November 16, 2006): 337–342.

4. H. Y. Cohen, C. Miller, K. J. Bitterman, N. R. Wall, et al., "Calorie restriction promotes mammalian cell survival by inducing the SIRT1 deacetylase," *Science* 305 (5682) (July 16, 2004): 390–2.

5. M. Lagouge, C. Argmann, Z. Gerhart-Hines, H. Meziane, et al., "Resveratrol improves mitochondrial function and protects against metabolic disease by activating SIRT1 and PGC-1α," *Cell* 127 (6) (December 15, 2006): 1091–1093.

6. J. A. Baur, K. J. Pearson, N. L. Price, H. A. Jamieson, et al., "Resveratrol improves health and survival of mice on a high-calorie diet," *Nature* 444 (7117) (November 16, 2006): 337–342.

7. N. Wade, "Red wine ingredient increases endurance, study shows," *New York Times,* November 17, 2006.

8. J. Baur and D. Sinclair, "Therapeutic potential of resveratrol: the *in vivo* evidence," *Nature Reviews Drug Discovery* 5 (June 2006): 493–505.

9. Y. Wang, K. W. Lee, F. L. Chan, S. Chen, et al., "The red wine polyphenol resveratrol displays bilevel inhibition on aromatase in breast cancer cells," *Toxicological Sciences* 92 (1) (2006): 71–77.

CHAPTER 8: LEAPS OF FAITH

1. Diane K. Hartle, Ph.D., Phillip Greenspan, Ph.D., and James L. Hargrove, Ph.D, *Muscadine Medicine,* Blue Heron Nutraceuticals, LLC, 2005.

2. P. Greenspan, J. D. Bauer, S. H. Pollock, J. D. Gangemi, E. P. Mayer,

A. Ghaffar, J. L. Hargrove and D. K. Hartle, "Anti-inflammatory properties of the muscadine grape (*Vitis rotundifolia*)." *Journal of Agricultural and Food Chemistry* 53 (2005): 8481-8484.

3. LeBlanc, M. R., "Cultivar, juice extraction, ultra violet irradiation and storage influence the stilbene content of Muscadine grape (*Vitis rotundifolia* Michx.). Ph.D. dissertation, Department of Horticulture, Louisiana State University, Baton Rouge, May 2006.

4. Langcake, P. "Disease resistance of *Vitis* spp. and the production of the stress metabolites resveratrol, epsilon-viniferin, alpha-viniferin and pterostilbene." *Physiological and Molecular Plant Pathology* 18 (1981): 213–226.

5. Langcake, P. and R. J. Pryce. "The production of resveratrol by *Vitis vinifera* and other members of the Vitaceae as a response to infection or injury." *Physiological and Molecular Plant Pathology* 9 (1976): 77–86.

CHAPTER 9: LIVE LONGER, IMPROVE MEMORY, ENHANCE ENDURANCE, AND MORE

1. J. Baur and D. Sinclair, "Therapeutic potential of resveratrol: the *in vivo* evidence," *Nature Reviews Drug Discovery* 5 (June 2006): 493–505.

2. R. Klatz, www.worldhealth.net.

3. Lenny Guarente, *Ageless quest: one scientist's search for genes that prolong youth* (Cold Spring Harbor, NY: Cold Spring Harbor Laboratory Press, 2003).

4. D. Rotman, "The fountain of health: antiaging researchers could provide a powerful approach to treating the many diseases of old age," *Technology Review,* March 2006.

5. Barbara Walters, "Live to 150, can you do it?" April 1, 2008, www.abc news.go.com/Health/Longevity/story?id=4544003&page=1

6. E. Lerner, "Will you still need me, will you still feed me, when I'm a hundred and twenty-four?" *Medicine at Michigan,* winter 2000.

7. Richard Weindruch and Roy L. Walford, *The retardation of aging and disease by dietary restriction* (Springfield, IL: Charles C. Thomas Publisher, 1988).

8. R. Weindruch, "Calorie restriction and aging," *Scientific American* 274 (1) (January 1996): 46–52.

9. R. Weindruch, "The retardation of aging by caloric restriction: studies in rodents and primates," *Toxicologic Pathology* 24 (6) (November–December 1996): 742–745.

10. M. Lagouge, C. Argmann, Z. Gerhart-Hines, H. Meziane, et al., "Resveratrol improves mitochondrial function and protects against metabolic disease by activating SIRT1 and PGC-1α," *Cell* 127 (6) (December 15, 2006): 1109–1122.

11. J.Bost, J. M. Smoliga, K. M. Bost, and J. C. Maroon, "Three months oral supplementation of a unique polyphenol mixture improves physical and neurocognitive performance indicators in sedentary adults," presented at American College of Sports Medicine (ACSM) annual meeting, May 2008.

12. M. Sharma and Y. K. Gupta, "Chronic treatment with trans resveratrol prevents intracerebroventricular streptozotocin induced cognitive impairment and oxidative stress in rats," *Life Sciences* 71 (21) (October 11, 2002): 2489–2498.

13. ImPACT website, www.impacttest.com.

14. B. B. Aggarwal and S. Shishir, *Resveratrol in health and disease* (Boca Raton, FL: CRC Press, 2006).

CHAPTER 10: DIABETES

1. "National diabetes fact sheet," National Center for Chronic Disease Prevention and Health Promotion, www.cdc.gov/diabetes/pubs/estimates05.htm.

2. Jennie Brand-Miller, Kaye Foster-Powell, Stephan Colagiuri, and Alan W. Barclay, *The new glucose revolution for diabetes* (New York: Marlowe & Company, 2007).

3. L. Barclay, "Growing evidence links resveratrol to extended life span," *Life Extension,* March 2007.

4. R. Rubin, "Diabetics face risk on drug choices," *USA Today,* June 4, 2007.

5. S. E. Nissen and K. Wolski, "Effect of rosiglitazone on the risk of myocardial infarction and death from cardiovascular causes," *New England Journal of Medicine* 356 (24) (June 14, 2007): 2457–2471.

6. J. Avorn, "Dangerous deception—hiding the evidence of adverse drug effects," *New England Journal of Medicine* 355 (21) (November 23, 2006): 2169–2171.

7. C. S. Hii and S. L. Howell, "Effects of flavonoids on insulin secretion and 45Ca2+ handling in rat islets of Langerhans," *Journal of Endocrinology* 107 (1) (October 1985): 1–8.

8. M. Vessal, M. Hemmati, and M. Vasei, "Antidiabetic effects of quercetin in streptozocin-induced diabetic rats," *Comparative Biochemistry and Physiology—Part C: Toxicology & Pharmacology* 135C (3) (July 2003): 357–364.

9. N. Al-Awwadi, J. Axay, P. Poucheret, G. Cassanas, et al., "Antidiabetic activity of red wine polyphenolic extract, ethanol, or both in streptozotocin-treated rats," *Journal of Agricultural and Food Chemistry* 52 (4) (February 25, 2004): 1008–1016.

10. E. Tsiani, D. Breen, and E. Park, "Resveratrol, a red wine polyphenol,

stimulates glucose but inhibits amino acid uptake and thymidine incorporation in L6 rat skeletal muscle cells," presented at the 66th Scientific Sessions of the American Diabetes Association (ADA), Washington, DC, June 2006.

11. E. Tsiani, D. Breen, and E. Park, "Cabernet or chardonnay: resveratrol prevents free fatty acid (FFA)–induced insulin resistance in parallel with prevention of FFA-induced increase in serine (307) phosphorylation of insulin receptor substrate 1 in skeletal muscle," presented at the 66th Scientific Sessions of the American Diabetes Association (ADA), Washington, DC, June 2006.

12. H. C. Su, L. M. Hung, and J. K. Chen, "Resveratrol, a red wine antioxidant, possesses an insulin-like effect in streptozotocin-induced diabetic rats," *American Journal of Physiology, Endocrinology and Metabolism* 290 (6) (June 2006): E1339–1346.

13. Sirtris Pharmaceuticals, Inc., http://investing.businessweek.com/research/stocks/private/snapshot.asp?privcapId=11420379

14. S. Sameer, S. K. Kulkarni, and K. Chopra, "Effect of resveratrol, a polyphenolic phytoalexin, on thermal hyperalgesia in a mouse model of diabetic neuropathic pain," *Fundamental & Clinical Pharmacology* 21 (1) (February 2007): 89–94.

CHAPTER 11: CARDIO PROTECTION

1. J. B. Herrick, "Clinical features of sudden obstruction of coronary arteries," *Journal of the American Medical Association* 59 (1912): 2015–2020.

2. G. K. Hansson, "Inflammation, atherosclerosis, and coronary artery disease," *New England Journal of Medicine* 352 (16) (April 21, 2005): 1685–1695.

3. F. Martin-Nizard, S. Sahpaz, C. Furman, J. Fruchart, et al., "Natural phenylpropanoids protect endothelial cells against oxidized LDL-induced cytotoxicity," *Planta Medica* 69 (3) (March 2003): 207–211.

4. S. V. Nigdikar, N. R. Williams, B. A. Griffin, and A. N. Howard, "Consumption of red wine polyphenols reduces the susceptibility of low-density lipoproteins to oxidation in vivo," *American Journal of Clinical Nutrition* 68 (2) (August 1998): 258–265.

5. E. B. Rimm, A. Klatsky, D. Grobbee, and M. J. Stampfer, "Review of moderate alcohol consumption and reduced risk of coronary heart disease: is the effect due to beer, wine, or spirits?," *British Medical Journal* 312 (7033) (March 23, 1996): 731–736.

6. G. Cao and R. L. Prior, "Red wine in moderation: potential health benefits independent of alcohol," *Nutrition in Clinical Care* 3 (2) (March–April 2000): 76–82.

7. M. H. Criqui and B. L. Ringel, "Does diet or alcohol explain the French paradox?" *Lancet* 344 (8939–8940) (December 24–31, 1994): 1719–1723.

8. A. Kasdallah-Grissa, B. Mornagui, M. Hammami, N. Ghardi, et al., "Protective effect of resveratrol on ethanol-induced lipid peroxidation in rats," *Alcohol and Alcoholism* 41 (3) (May–June 2006): 236–239.

9. Y. Meng, Q. Y. Ma, X. P. Kou, and J. Xu, "Effect of resveratrol on activation of nuclear factor kappa-B and inflammatory factors in rat model of acute pancreatitis," *World Journal of Gastroenterology* 11 (4) (January 28, 2005): 525–528.

10. Y. J. Surh, K. S. Chun, H. H. Cha, S. S. Han, et al., "Molecular mechanisms underlying chemopreventive activities of anti-inflammatory phytochemicals: down-regulation of COX-2 and iNOS through suppression of NF-kappa B activation," *Mutation Research* 480–481 (September 1, 2001): 243–268.

11. F. Yeung, J. E. Hoberg, C. S. Ramsey, M. D. Keller, et al., "Modulation of NF-κB-dependent transcription and cell survival by the SIRT1 deacetylase," *EMBO Journal* 23 (12) (June 16, 2004): 2369–2380.

12. Z. Wang, Y. Huang, J. Zou, K. Cao, et al., "Effects of red wine and wine polyphenol resveratrol on platelet aggregation in vivo and in vitro," *International Journal of Molecular Medicine* 9 (1) (January 2002): 77–79.

13. J. G. Keevil, H. E. Osman, J. D. Reed, and J. D. Folts, "Grape juice, but not orange juice or grapefruit juice, inhibits human platelet aggression," *Journal of Nutrition* 130 (1) (January 2000): 53–56.

14. R. I. Kirk, J. A. Deitch, J. M. Wu, and K. M. Lerea, "Resveratrol decreases early signaling events in washed platelets but has little effect on platelet aggregation in whole blood," *Blood Cells, Molecules and Diseases* 26 (2) (April 2000): 144–150.

15. B. Olas and B. Wachowicz, "Resveratrol, a phenolic antioxidant with effects on blood platelet functions," *Platelets* 16 (5) (August 2005): 251–260.

16. C. R. Pace-Asciak, S. Hahn, E. P. Diamandis, G. Soleas, et al., "The red wine phenolics trans-resveratrol and quercetin block human platelet aggregation and eicosanoid synthesis: implications for protection against coronary heart disease," *Clinica Chimica Acta* 235 (2) (March 31, 1995): 207–219.

17. C. R. Pace-Asciak, O. Rounova, S. E. Hahn, E. P. Diamandis, et al. "Wines and grape juices as modulators of platelet aggregation in healthy human subjects," *Clinica Chimica Acta* 246 1996 (1–2) (March 15, 1996): 163–182.

18. M. Seigneur, J. Bonnet, B. Dorian, et al., "Effect of the consumption of alcohol, white wine, and red wine on platelet function and serum lipids," *Journal of Applied Cardiology* 5 (3) (1990): 215–222.

19. S. Shigematsu, S. Ishida, M. Hara, M. Takahashi, et al., "Resveratrol, a red wine constituent polyphenol, prevents superoxide-dependent inflammatory responses induced by ischemia/reperfusion, platelet-activating factor, or oxidants," *Free Radical Biology and Medicine* 34 (7) (April 1, 2003): 810–817.

20. G. Stef, A. Csiszar, K. Lerea, Z. Ungvari, et al., "Resveratrol inhibits aggregation of platelets from high-risk cardiac patients with aspirin resistance," *Journal of Cardiovascular Pharmacology* 48 (2) (August 2006): 1–5.

21. J. A. Vita, "Polyphenols and cardiovascular disease: effects on endothelial and platelet functions," *American Journal of Clinical Nutrition* 81 (1 supplement) (January 2005): 292S–297S.

22. P. Pignatelli, F. M. Pulcinelli, A. Celestini, L. Lenti, et al., "The flavonoids quercetin and catechin synergistically inhibit platelet function by antagonizing the intracellular production of hydrogen peroxide," *American Journal of Clinical Nutrition* 72 (5) (November 2000): 1150–1155.

23. J. B. Pillai, A. Isbatan, S. Imai, and M. P. Gupta, "Poly(ADP-ribose) polymerase-1-dependent cardiac myocyte cell death during heart failure is mediated by NAD^+ depletion and reduced $Sir2\alpha$ deacetylase activity," *Journal of Biological Chemistry* 280 (52) (December 30, 2005): 43121–43130.

24. K. Bezstarosti, S. Das, J. M. Lamers, and D. K. Das, "Differential proteomic profiling to study the mechanism of cardiac pharmacological preconditioning by resveratrol," *Journal of Cellular and Molecular Medicine* 10 (4) (October–December 2006): 896–907.

25. C. H. R. Wallace, I. Baczkó, L. Jones, M. Fercho, et al., "Inhibition of cardiac voltage-gated sodium channels by grape polyphenols," *British Journal of Pharmacology* 149 (6) (November 2006): 657–665.

26. M. H. Criqui, L. D. Cowan, H. A. Tyroler, S. Bangdiwala, et al. "Lipoproteins as mediators for the effects of alcohol consumption and cigarette smoking on cardiovascular mortality: results from the lipid research clinics follow-up study," *American Journal of Epidemiology* 126 (4) (October 1987): 629–637.

27. M. Corral-Debrinski, T. Horton, M. T. Lott, J. M. Shoffner, et al., "Mitochondrial DNA deletions in human brain: regional variability and increase with advanced age," *Nature Genetics* 2 (4) (December 1992): 324–329.

28. D. C. Wallace, "Mitochondrial diseases in man and mouse," *Science* 283 (5407) (March 5, 1999): 1482–1488.

29. E. S. Ford, D. R. Labarthe, U. A. Ajani, J. B. Croft, et al., "Explaining the decrease in U.S. deaths from coronary disease, 1980–2000," *New England Journal of Medicine* 356 (23) (June 7, 2007): 2388–2398.

30. P. S. Ray, G. Maulik, G. A. Cordis, A. A. Bertelli, et al., "The red wine an-

tioxidant resveratrol protects isolated rat hearts from ischemia reperfusion injury," *Free Radical Biology and Medicine* 27 (1–2) (July 1999): 160–169.

CHAPTER 12: THE ANTICANCER EFFECT

1. Ian F. Tannock, Richard P. Hill, Robert G. Bristow, and Lea Harrington, *The Basic Science of Oncology,* 4th ed. (New York: McGraw-Hill Companies, 2005).
2. *Cancer facts & figures 2007* (Atlanta: American Cancer Society, 2007).
3. M. Jang and J. M. Pezzuto, "Effects of resveratrol on 12-O-tetradecanoyl-phorbol-13-acetate-induced oxidative events and gene expression in mouse skin," *Cancer Letters* 134 (1) (December 11, 1998): 81–89.
4. M. Jang and J. M. Pezzuto, "Cancer chemopreventive activity of resveratrol," *Drugs under Experimental and Clinical Research* 25 (2–3) (1999): 65–77.
5. C. Yu, Y. G. Shin, J. W. Kosmeder, J. M. Pezzuto, et al., "Liquid chromatography/tandem mass spectrometric determination of inhibition of human cytochrome P450 isozymes by resveratrol and resveratrol-3-sulfate," *Rapid Communications in Mass Spectrometry* 17 (4) (2003) 307–313.
6. K. Bhat, J. W. Kosmeder, and J. M. Pezzuto, "Biological Effects of Resveratrol," *Antioxidants and Redox Signaling* 3 (6) (December 2001): 1041–1064.
7. B. Aggarwal, A. Bhardwaj, R. Aggarwal, N. Seeram, et al., "Role of resveratrol in prevention and therapy of cancer: preclinical and clinical studies," *Anticancer Research* 24 (5A) (September–October 2004): 2783–2840.
8. M. Asensi, I. Medina, A. Ortega, J. Carretero, et al., "Inhibition of cancer growth by resveratrol is related to its low bioavailability," *Free Radical Biology and Medicine* 33 (3) (August 1, 2002): 387–398.
9. M. Athar, J. H. Back, X. Tang, H. K. Kim, et al., "Resveratrol: a review of preclinical studies for human cancer prevention," *Toxicology and Applied Pharmacology* 224 (3) (November 1, 2007): 274–283.
10. M. H. Aziz, M. S. Reagan-Shaw, J. Wu, B. J. Longley, et al., "Chemoprevention of skin cancer by grape constituent resveratrol: relevance to human disease?" *FASEB Journal* 19 (9) (July 2005): 1193–1195.
11. S. Banerjee, C. Bueso-Ramos, and B. B. Aggarwal, "Suppression of 7,12-dimethylbenz(a)anthracene-induced mammary carcinogenesis in rats by resveratrol: role of nuclear factor-kappaB, cyclooxygenase 2, and matrix metalloprotease 9," *Cancer Research* 62 (17) (September 1, 2002): 4945–4954.
12. G. Berge, S. Øvrebø, E. Eilertsen, A. Haugen, et al., "Analysis of resvera-

trol as a lung cancer chemopreventive agent in A/J mice exposed to benzo[a]pyrene," *British Journal of Cancer* 91 (7) (October 4, 2004): 1380–1383.

13. K. P. Bhat, D. Lantvit, K. Christov, R. G. Mehta, et al., "Estrogenic and antiestrogenic properties of resveratrol in mammary tumor models," *Cancer Research* 61 (20) (October 15, 2001): 7456–7463.

14. D. J. Boocock, D. E. Brenner, A. J. Gescher, W. P. Steward, et al., "Phase I repeat-dose clinical study of safety, pharmacokinetics and pharmaco-dynamics of resveratrol," NCI Division of Cancer Prevention, N01-CN-25025, protocol version 32.

15. D. J. Boocock, G. E. Faust, K. R. Patel, A. M. Schinas, et al., "Phase I dose escalation pharmacokinetic study in healthy volunteers of resveratrol, a potential cancer chemopreventive agent," *Cancer Epidemiology, Bio-markers and Prevention* 16 (6) (June 2007): 1246–1252.

16. K. Bove, D. W. Lincoln, and M. F. Tsan, "Effect of resveratrol on growth of 4T1 breast cancer cells in vitro and in vivo," *Biochemical and Biophysi-cal Research Communications* 291 (4) (March 8, 2002): 1001–1005.

17. G. Cowley, "Cancer and diet: can you eat to beat malignancy?," *News-week,* November 30, 1998.

18. R. H. Dashwood, "Frontiers in polyphenols and cancer prevention," *Journal of Nutrition* 137 (1 supplement) (January 2007): 267S–269S.

19. S. G. Elias, P. Peeters, D. E. Grobbee, and P. A. van Noord, "Transient caloric restriction and cancer risk (The Netherlands)," *Cancer Causes Control* 18 (1) (February 2007): 1–5.

20. T. Fotis, M. S. Pepper, E. Atkas, S. Briet, et al., "Flavonoids, dietary-derived inhibitors of cell proliferation and in vitro angiogenesis," *Can-cer Research* 57 (14) (July 15, 1997): 2916–2921.

21. Z. D. Fu., Y. Cao, K. F. Wang, S. F. Xu, et al., "Chemopreventive effect of resveratrol to cancer," *Ai Zheng* 23 (8) (August 2004): 869–873.

22. S. Garvin, K. Ollinger, and C. Dabrosin, "Resveratrol induces apoptosis and inhibits angiogenesis in human breast cancer xenografts in vivo," *Cancer Letters* 231 (1) (January 8, 2006): 113–122.

23. A. J. Gescher and W. P. Steward, "Relationship between mechanisms, bioavailability, and preclinical chemopreventive efficacy of resveratrol: a conundrum," *Cancer Epidemiology, Biomarkers and Prevention* 12 (10) (October 2003): 933–957.

24. C. E. Harper, B. B. Patel, J. Wang, A. Arabshahi, et al., "Resveratrol sup-presses prostate cancer progression in transgenic mice," *Carcinogene-sis* 28 (9) (September 2007): 1946–1953.

25. S. D. Hursting, J. A. Lavigne, D. Berrigan, S. N. Perkins, et al., "Calorie restriction, aging, and cancer prevention: mechanisms of action and ap-plicability to humans," *Annual Review of Medicine* 54 (2003): 131–152.

26. K. Igura, T. Ohta, Y. Kuroda, and K. Kaji, "Resveratrol and quercetin inhibit angiogenesis in vitro," *Cancer Letters* 171 (1): (September 28, 2001): 11–16.
27. M. Jang, L. Cai, G. O. Udeani, K. V. Slowing, et al., "Cancer chemopreventive activity of resveratrol, a natural product derived from grapes," *Science* 275 (5297) (January 10, 1997): 218–220.
28. R. Lu and G. Serrero, "Resveratrol, a natural product derived from grape, exhibits antiestrogenic activity and inhibits the growth of human breast cancer cells," *Journal of Cellular Physiology* 179 (3) (June 1999): 297–304.
29. R. M. Niles, M. B. McFarland, A. Weimer, Y. M. Redkar, et al., "Resveratrol is a potent inducer of apoptosis in human melanoma cells," *Cancer Letters* 190 (2) (February 20, 2003): 157–163.
30. B. Schneider, D. Fischer, S. Coelho, F. Roussi, et al., "(Z)-3,5,4'-Tri-O-methyl-resveratrol induces apoptosis in human lymphoblastoid cells independently of their p53 status," *Cancer Letters* 211 (2) (August 10, 2004): 155–161.
31. T. Whitsett, M. Carpenter, and C. A. Lamartiniere, "Resveratrol, but not EGCG, in the diet suppresses DMBA-induced mammary cancer in rats," *Journal of Carcinogenesis* 5 (May 15, 2006): 15.
32. W. Sun, W. Wang, J. Kim, P. Keng, et al., "Anti-cancer effect of resveratrol is associated with induction of apoptosis via a mitochondrial pathway alignment," *Advances in Experimental Medicine and Biology* 614 (2008): 179–186.
33. Y. Schneider, F. Vincent, B. Duranton, L. Badolo, et al., "Anti-proliferative effect of resveratrol, a natural component of grapes and wine, on human colonic cancer cells," *Cancer Letters* 158 (1) (September 29, 2000): 85–91.

CHAPTER 13: STROKE PREVENTION

1. H. Inoue, X. F. Ziang, T. Katayama, S. Osada, et al., "Brain protection by resveratrol and fenofibrate against stroke requires peroxisome proliferator-activated receptor alpha in mice," *Neuroscience Letters* 352 (3) (December 11, 2003): 203–206.
2. H. Zhuang, Y. S. Kim, R. C. Koehler, and S. Doré, "Potential mechanism by which resveratrol, a red wine constituent, protects neurons," *Annuals of the New York Academy of Sciences* 993 (May 2003): 276–286.
3. K. Mizutani, K. Ikeda, Y. Kawai, and Y. Yamori, "Protective effect of resveratrol on oxidative damage in male and female stroke-prone spontaneously hypertensive rats," *Clinical and Experimental Pharmacology and Physiology* 28 (1–2) (January–February 2001): 55–59.
4. K. J. Mukamal, A. Ascherio, M. A. Mittleman, K. M. Conigrave, et al., "Al-

cohol and risk for ischemic stroke in men: the role of drinking patterns and usual beverage," *Annuals of Internal Medicine* 142 (1) (January 4, 2005): 11–19.

5. K. Sinha, G. Chaudhary, and Y. K. Gupta, "Protective effect of resveratrol against oxidative stress in middle cerebral artery occlusion model of stroke in rats," *Life Sciences* 71 (6) (June 28, 2002): 655–665.

6. O. Ates, S. Cayli, E. Altinoz, I. Gurses, et al., "Neuroprotection by resveratrol against traumatic brain injury in rats," *Molecular and Cellular Biochemistry* 294 (1–2) (January 2007): 137–144.

7. U. Kiziltepe, N. N. Turan, U. Han, A. T. Ulus, et al., "Resveratrol, a red wine polyphenol, protects spinal cord from ischemia-reperfusion injury," *Journal of Vascular Surgery* 40 (1) (July 2004): 138–145.

CHAPTER 14: DEGENERATIVE BRAIN DISEASES AND BRAIN PROTECTION

1. C. M. Carlsson, C. E. Gleason, and S. Asthana, "Update on diagnosis and treatment of Alzheimer disease," *Consultant Pharmacist* (2005): 77–88.

2. M. A. Smith, G. Perry, P. L. Richey, L. M. Sayre, et al., "Oxidative damage in Alzheimer's," *Nature* 382 (6587) (July 11, 1996): 120–121.

3. D. Weisman, E. Hakimian, and G. J. Ho, "Interleukins, inflammation, and mechanisms of Alzheimer's disease," *Vitamins and Hormones* 74 (2006): 505–530.

4. V. M. Ingram, "Alzheimer's disease," *American Scientist* 91 (4) (July–August 2003): 312.

5. D. Kim, M. D. Nguyen, M. M. Dobbin, A. Fischer, et al. "SIRT1 deacetylase protects against neurodegeneration in models for Alzheimer's disease and amyotrophic lateral sclerosis," *EMBO Journal* 26 (13) (July 11, 2007): 3169–3179.

6. P. Marambaud, H. Zhao, and P. Davies, "Resveratrol promotes clearance of Alzheimer's disease amyloid-B peptides," *Journal of Biological Chemistry* 280 (45) (November 11, 2005): 37377–37382.

7. T. S. Anekonda, "Resveratrol—a boon for treating Alzheimer's disease?," *Brain Research Reviews* 52 (2) (September 2006): 316–326.

8. M. S. Wolf, "Shutting down Alzheimer's," *Scientific American* 294 (5) (May 2006): 72–79.

9. R. C. Adelman, "The Alzheimerization of aging: a brief update," *Experimental Gerontology* 33 (1–2) (January–March 1998): 155–157.

10. W. E. Klunk, H. Engler, A. Nordberg, Y. Wang, et al., "Imaging brain amyloid in Alzheimer's disease with Pittsburgh Compound-B," *Annals of Neurology* 55 (3) (March 2004): 306–319.

11. C. Rosano and A. B. Newman, "Cardiovascular disease and risk of

Alzheimer's disease," *Neurological Research* 28 (6) (September 2006): 612–620.

12. E. R. Rosick, "The deadly link between heart disease and Alzheimer's," *Life Extension,* June 2007.

13. A. Russo. M. Palumbo, C. Aliano, L. Lempereur, et al., "Red wine micronutrients as protective agents in Alzheimer-like induced insult," *Life Sciences* 72 (21) (April 11, 2003): 2369–2379.

14. M. Sastre, T. Klockgether, and M. T. Heneka, "Contribution of inflammatory process to Alzheimer's disease: molecular mechanisms," *International Journal of Developmental Neuroscience* 24 (2–3) (April–May 2006): 167–176.

15. X. Sun, G. He, H. Qing, W. Zhou, et al., "Hypoxia facilitates Alzheimer's disease pathogenesis by up-regulating BACE1 gene expression," *Proceedings of the National Academy of Sciences of the United States of America* 103 (49) (December 5, 2006): 18727–18732.

16. "DHA (docosahexaenoic acid), an omega-3 fatty acid, is slowing the progression of Alzheimer's disease," www.clinicaltrials.gov.

17. "Guarente shows increased SIRT1 expression improves 'quality of life' in Huntington's mouse model," www.biomol.com/About_Us/BIOMOL_News/BIOMOL_Newswire/BIOMOL_Newswire_Archives/210/?vobId=995&pm=326, April 1, 2008.

18. J. T. Greenamyre, "Huntington's disease—making connections," *New England Journal of Medicine* 356 (5) (February 1, 2007): 518–520.

19. A. Russo, M. Palumbo, C. Aliano, L. Lempereur, et al., "Red wine micronutrients as protective agents in Alzheimer-like induced insult," *Life Sciences* 72 (21) (April 11, 2003): 2369–2379.

20. E. Savaskan, G. Olivieri, F. Meier, E. Seifritz, et al., "Red wine ingredient resveratrol protects from beta-amyloid neurotoxicity," *Gerontology* 49 (6) (November–December 2003): 380–383.

21. K. Schindlar, E. Ventura, T. S. Rex, P. Elliott, et al., "SIRT1 activation confers neuroprotection in experimental optic neurtis," *Investigative Ophthalmology and Visual Science* 48 (8) (August 2007): 3602–3609.

CHAPTER 15: OTHER INFLAMMATORY CONDITIONS

1. S. S. An, T. R. Bai, J. H. Bates, J. L. Black, et al., "Airway smooth muscle dynamics: a common pathway of airway obstruction in asthma," *European Respiratory Journal* 29 (5) (May 2007): 834–860.

2. L. E. Donnelly, R. Newton, G. E. Kennedy, P. S. Fenwick, et al., "Anti-inflammatory effects of resveratrol in lung epithelial cells: molecular mechanisms," *American Journal of Physiology Lung Cellular Molecular Physiology* 287 (4) (October 2004) 774–783.

3. S. V. Culpitt, D. F. Rogers, P. S. Fenwick, P. Shah, et al., "Inhibition by red wine extract, resveratrol, of cytokine release by alveolar macrophages in COPD," *Thorax* 58 (11) (November 2003): 942–946.

4. Y. Schneider, F. Vincent, B. Duranton, L. Badolo, et al., "Anti-proliferative effect of resveratrol, a natural component of grapes and wine, on human colonic cancer cells," *Cancer Letters* 158 (1) (September 29, 2000): 85–91.

5. A. R. Martín, I. Villegas, C. La Casa, and C. A. de la Lastra, "Resveratrol, a polyphenol found in grapes, suppresses oxidative damage and stimulates apoptosis during early colonic inflammation in rats," *Biochemical Pharmacology* 67 (7) (April 1, 2004): 1399–1410.

6. A. R. Martín, I. Villegas, M. Sánchez-Hidalgo, and C. A. de la Lastra, "The effects of resveratrol, a phytoalexin derived from red wines, on chronic inflammation induced in an experimentally induced colitis model," *British Journal of Pharmacology* 147 (8) (April 2006): 873–885.

7. P. Castilla, R. Echarri, A. Davalos, E. Cerrato, et al., "Concentrated red grape juice exerts antioxidant, hypolipidemic, and antiimflammatory effects in both hemodialysis patients and healthy subjects," *American Journal of Clinical Nutrition* 84 (1) (July 2006): 252–262.

8. V. Chander, N. Tirkey, and K. Chopra, "Resveratrol, a polyphenolic phytoalexin, protects against cyclosporine-induced nephrotoxicity through nitric oxide dependent mechanism," *Toxicology* 210 (1) (May 15, 2005): 55–64.

9. N. Elmali, I. Esenkaya, A. Harma, K. Ertem, et al., "Effect of resveratrol in experimental osteoarthritis in rabbits," *Inflammation Research* (4) (April 2005): 158–162.

10. N. Elmali, O. Baysal, A. Harma, I. Esenkaya, et al., "Effects of resveratrol in inflammatory arthritis," *Inflammation* 30 (1–2) (April 2007) 1–6.

11. J. B. Johnson, W. Summer, R. G. Cutler, B. Martin, et al., "Alternate day calorie restriction improves clinical findings and reduces markers of oxidative stress and inflammation in overweight adults with moderate asthma," *Free Radical Biology and Medicine* 42 (5) (March 1, 2007): 665–674.

12. M. A. Birrell, K. McCluskie, S. Wong, L. E. Donnelly, et al., "Resveratrol, an extract of red wine, inhibits lipopolysaccharide induced airway neutrophilia and inflammatory mediators through an NF-κB-independent mechanism," *FASEB Journal* 19 (7) (May 2005): 840–841.

13. Y. Meng, Q. Y. Ma, X. P. Kou, and J. Xu, "Effect of resveratrol on activation of nuclear factor κ-B and inflammatory factors in rat model of acute pancreatitis," *World Journal of Gastroenterology* 11 (4) (January 28, 2005): 525–528.

CHAPTER 16: SOURCES, SAFETY, BIOAVAILABILITY, AND DOSAGE

1. D. M. Goldberg, J. Yan, and G. J. Soleas, "Absorption of three wine-related polyphenols in three different matrices by healthy subjects," *Chemical Biochemistry* 36 (1) (February 2003): 79–87.

2. J. F. Marier, P. Vachon, A. Gritsas, J. Zhang, et al., "Metabolism and disposition of resveratrol in rats: extent of absorption, glucuronidation, and enterohepatic recirculation evidenced by a linked-rat model," *Journal of Pharmacology and Experimental Therapeutics* 302 (1) (July 2002) 369–373.

3. G. J. Soleas, M. Angelini, I. Grass, E. P. Diamandis, et al., "Absorption of trans-resveratrol in rats," *Methods in Enzymology* 335 (2001): 145–154.

4. G. J. Soleas, J. Yan, and D. M. Goldberg, "Measurement of trans-resveratrol, (+)-catechin, and quercetin in rat and human blood and urine by gas chromatography with mass selective detection," *Methods in Enzymology* 335 (2001): 130–145.

5. T. Walle, F. Hsieh, M. H. DeLegge, J. E. Oatis, et al., "High absorption but very low bioavailability of oral resveratrol in humans," *Drug Metabolism and Disposition* 32 (12) (December 2004): 1377–1382.

6. D. J. Boocock, D. E. Brenner, A. J. Gescher, W. P. Steward, et al., "Phase I repeat-dose clinical study of safety, pharmacokinetics and pharmacodynamics of resveratrol," NCI Division of Cancer Prevention, N01-CN-25025, protocol version 32.

7. D. J. Boocock, A. J. Gescher, V. Brown, and G. E. Faust, "Phase I single-dose safety and pharmacokinetics clinical study of the potential cancer chemopreventive agent resveratrol," abstract 5741, *Proceedings of the American Association for Cancer Research* 47 (2006).

8. D. J. Boocock, G. Faust, K. R. Patel, A. M. Schinas, et al., "Phase I dose escalation pharmacokinetic study in healthy volunteers of resveratrol, a potential cancer chemopreventive agent," *Cancer Epidemiology, Biomarkers, and Prevention* 16 (6) (June 2007): 1246–1252.

9. J. Dudley and D. Das, "Resveratrol, a polyphenolic antioxidant in red wine, is dose-dependent in delivering cardioprotection," *Experimental Biology 2007: Meeting Abstracts* 114 (5).

10. Y. H. Feng, W. L. Zhou, O. L. Wu, X. Y. Li, et al., "Low dose of resveratrol enhanced immune response of mice," *Acta Pharmacologica Sinica* 23 (10) (October 2002): 893–897.

11. M. Fenech, "Nutritional treatment of genome instability: a paradigm shift in disease prevention and in the setting of recommended dietary allowances," *Nutrition Research Reviews* 16 (1) (June 2003): 109–122.

12. M. E. Juan, M. B. Vinardell, and J. M. Planas, "The daily oral administra-

tion of high doses of trans-resveratrol to rats for 28 days is not harmful," *Journal of Nutrition* 132 (2) February 2002: 257–260.

13. M. Athar, J. H. Back, X. Tang, H. K. Kim, et al., "Resveratrol: A review of preclinical studies for human cancer prevention," *Toxicology and Applied Pharmacology* 224 (3) (November 1, 2007): 274–283.

14. J. A. Crowell, B. J. Korytko, R. L. Morrissey, T. D. Booth, et al., "Resveratrol-associated renal toxicity," *Toxicological Sciences* 82 (2) (December 2004): 614–619.

15. M. Floreani, E. Napoli, L. Quintieri, and P. Palatini, "Oral administration of trans-resveratrol to guinea pigs increases cardiac DT-diaphorase and catalase activities, and protects isolated atria from menadione toxicity," *Life Sciences* 72 (24) (May 2, 2003): 2741–2750.

16. L. Frame, R. Hart, and J. Leakey, "Caloric restriction as a mechanism mediating resistance to environmental disease," based on presentation at the Third BELLE Conference on Toxicological Defense Mechanisms and the Shape of Dose-Response Relationships, November 12–14 1996, Research Triangle Park, NC.

17. V. Hebbar, G. Shen, R. Hu, B. R. Kim, et al., "Toxicogenomics of resveratrol in rat liver," *Life Sciences* 76 (20) (April 1, 2005): 2299–2314.

18. S. Masten and K. E. Haneke, "Trans-resveratrol [501-36-0]: review of toxicological literature," National Institute of Environmental Health Sciences, March 2002.

19. H. Zhang, C. Dou, and F. Gu, "Advances in the study on pharmacological actions of *Polygonum cuspidatum Sieb. et Zucc.:* clearing heat and detoxication," *Zhong Yao Cai* (*Journal of Chinese Medicinal Materials*) 26 (8) (August 2003): 606–610.

Tea

20. Cao G. Sofic E. and R. L. Prior, "Antioxidant capacity of tea and common vegetables," *Journal of Agricultural and Food Chemistry* 44 (11) (November 1996): 3426–3431.

21. HN Graham, "Green tea composition, consumption, and polyphenol chemistry," *Preventive Medicine* 21 (3) May 1992: 334–350

22. A. Josephs, "Antioxidant superstars resveratrol and green tea backed by National Cancer Institute," National Cancer Institute fact sheet, November 27, 2002.

23. A. Conte, S. Pellegrini, and D. Tagliazucchi, "Synergestic protection of PC12 cells from beta-amyloid toxicity by resveratrol and catechin," *Brain Research Bulletin* 62 (1) (November 15, 2003): 29–38.

24. S. E. Ebeler, C. A. Brenneman, G. Kim, W. T. Jewell, et al., "Dietary catechin delays tumor onset in a transgenic mouse model," *American Journal of Clinical Nutrition* 76 (4) (October 2002): 865–872.

25. P. Strobel, C. Allard, T. Perez-Acle, R. Calderon, et al., "Myricetin, quercetin and catechin-gallate inhibit glucose uptake in isolated rat adipocytes," *Biochemical Journal* 386 (Pt. 3) (March 15, 2005): 471–478.

26. M. B. Hicks, Y. H. P. Hsieh, and L. N. Bell. "Tea preparation and its influence on methylxanthine concentration," *Food Research International* 29 (3–4) (April–May 1996): 325–330.

27. H. R. Lieberman, "The effects of ginseng, ephedrine, and caffeine on cognitive performance, mood and energy," *Nutrition Reviews* 59 (4) (April 2001): 91–102.

28. Bennett Alan Weinberg and Bonnie K. Bealer, *The world of caffeine: the science and culture of the world's most popular drug* (New York: Routledge, 2001).

29. K. C. Wilson and M. N. Clifford, *Tea: cultivation to consumption* New York: Chapman and Hall, 1992).

30. M. A. Bokuchava and N. I. Skobeleva, "The biochemistry and technology of tea manufacture," *Critical Reviews in Food Science and Nutrition* 12 (4) (1980): 303–370.

Apples and Other Fruit

31. R. H. Liu, "Health benefits of fruit and vegetables are from additive and synergistic combinations of phytochemicals," *American Journal of Clinical Nutrition* 78 supplement (3) (September 2003): 517S–520S.

32. M. V. Eberhard, C. Y. Lee, and R. H. Liu, "Antioxidant activity of fresh apples," *Nature* 405 (6789) (June 22, 2000): 903–904.

33. J. Sun, Y. F. Chu, X. Wu, and R. H. Liu, "Antioxidant and antiproliferative activities of common fruits," *Journal of Agricultural and Food Chemistry* 50 (25) (December 4, 2002): 7449–7954.

34. Y. F. Chu, J. Sun, X. Wu, and R. H. Liu, "Antioxidant and antiproliferative activities of vegetables," *Journal of Agricultural and Food Chemistry* 50 (23) (November 6, 2002): 6910–6916.

35. E. J. Rogers, S. Milhalik, D. Orthiz, and T. B. Shea, "Apple juice prevents oxidative stress and impaired cognitive performance caused by genetic and dietary deficiencies in mice," *Journal of Health, Nutrition and Aging* 8 (2) (2004): 92–97.

36. F. Tchantchou, M. Graves, D. Ortiz, E. Rogers, et al., "Dietary supplementation with apple juice concentrate alleviates the compensatory increase in glutathione synthase transcription and activity that accompanies dietary- and genetically-induced oxidative stress," *Journal of Health, Nutrition and Aging* 8 (6) (2004): 492–496.

Chocolate

37. A. Scalbert and G. Williamson, "Chocolate: modern science investigates an ancient medicine: dietary intake and bioavailability of polyphenols," *Journal of Nutrition* 130: 2073S–2085S.

38. A. Scalbert, I. T. Johnson, and M. Saltmarsh, "Polyphenols: antioxidants and beyond," *American Journal of Clinical Nutrition* 81 (supplement) (January 2005): 215S–217S.

39. D. Taubert, R. Berkels, R. Roecen, and W. Klavs, "Dark chocolate and blood pressure in elderly individuals with isolated systolic hypertension," *Journal of the American Medical Association* 290 (8) (August 27, 2003): 989–1118.

40. D. Taubert, R. Roesen, C. Lehmann, N. Jung, et al., "Effects of low habitual cocoa intake on blood pressure and bioactive nitric oxide: a randomized controlled trial," *Journal of the American Medical Association* 298 (1) (July 4, 2007): 49–60.

41. P. Pasqualetti, G. Desideri, D. Grassi, S. Necozione, et al., "Cocoa reduces blood pressure and insulin resistance and improves endothelium-dependent vasodilation in hypertensives," *Hypertension* 46 (2) (August 1, 2005): 398–405.

42. C. L. Keen, "Chocolate: food as a medicine/medicine as food," *Journal of the American College of Nutrition* 20 (Supplement) (October 2001): 436S–439S, 440S–442S.

43. M. Diebolt, B. Bucher, and R. Andriantsitohaina, "Wine polyphenols decrease blood pressure, improve NO vasodilatation, and induce gene expression," *Hypertension* 38 (2) (August 2001): 159–165.

44. R. R. Holt, S. A. Lazarus, M. C. Sullards, Q. Y. Zhu, et al., "Procyanidin dimer B2 [epicatechin-(4β-8)-epicatechin] in human plasma after the consumption of a flavanol-rich cocoa," *American Journal of Clinical Nutrition* 76 (4) (October 2002): 798–804.

45. M. B. Engler, M. M. Engler, C. Y. Chen, M. J. Malloy, et al., "Flavonoid-rich dark chocolate improves endothelial function and increases plasma epicatechin concentrations in healthy adults," *Journal of the American College of Nutrition* 23 (3) (June 2004): 197–204.

46. D. Rein, T. G. Paglieroni, D. A. Pearson, T. Wun, et al., "Cocoa and wine polyphenols modulate platelet activation and function," *Journal of Nutrition* 130 (8S supplement) (August 2000): 2120S–2126S.

47. R. M. Lamuela-Raventós, A. I. Romero-Pérez, C. Andres-Licueva, and A. Tornero, "Review: health effects of cocoa flavonoids," *Food Science and Technology International*, 11 (3) (June 1, 2005): 159–176.

Websites

48. www.biotivia.com
49. www.revgenetics.com
50. www.longevinex.com
51. www.revatrol.com
52. www.resvinatrolcomplete.com
53. www.lifetimevitamins.com

Powergrape References

54. S. Lafay, "The grape extract rich in procyanidins which reduce exercise-induced oxidative stress of professional soccer players," poster, Third Congress on Polyphenols, Malta, 2006.
55. S. Lafay, "Whole grape extract reduces exercise-induced oxidative stress of professional athletes," Powergrape, poster 258, Conference on Polyphenols and Health, Kyoto, November 2007.
56. Powergrape press release, Berkem, March 6, 2007, www.berkem.com.
57. J. L. Barger, T. Kayo, J. M. Vann, E. B. Arias, et al., "A low dose of dietary resveratrol partially mimics caloric restriction and retards aging parameters in mice," *PLoS ONE* 3 (6) (June 4, 2008): e2264.

CHAPTER 17: THE HOWS AND WHYS OF OVERWEIGHT

1. A. Hilbert, W. Rief, and E. Braehler, "Stigmatizing attitudes toward obesity in a representative population-based sample," *Obesity* 16 (7) (July 2008): 1529–1534.
2. N. A. Christakis and J. H. Fowler, "The spread of obesity in a large social network over 32 years," *New England Journal of Medicine* 357 (4) (July 26, 2007): 370–379.
3. USA Today Weight-loss Challenge, www.usatoday.com/news/health/weightloss/default.htm
4. K-T Ayoob, R. L. Duyff, and D. Quagliani, "Position of the American Dietetic Association: food and nutrition misinformation," *Journal of the American Dietetic Association* 102 (2) (February 2002): 260–266.
5. H. Klüver and P. C. Bucy, "Preliminary analysis of functions of the temporal lobes in monkeys," *Archives of Neurology and Psychiatry* 42 (1939): 979–1000.
6. R. Lilly, J. L. Cummings, D. F. Benson, and M. Frankel, "The human Klüver-Bucy syndrome," *Neurology* 33 (9) (September 1983): 1141–1145.
7. B. M. Kuehn, "Brain scans, genes provide addiction clues," *Journal of the American Medical Association* 297 (13) (April 4, 2007): 1419–1421.

CHAPTER 18: WHAT'S A PERSON TO DO?

1. A. Y. Sun, A. Simonyi, and G. Y Sun, "The 'French Paradox' and beyond: neuroprotective effects of polyphenols," *Free Radical Biology and Medicine* 32 (4) (February 15, 2002): 314–318.

2. J. A. Vita, "Polyphenols and cardiovascular disease: effects on endothelial and platelet functions," *American Journal of Clinical Nutrition* 81(1) (January 2005): 292S–297S.

3. Y. Wang, K. W. Lee, F. L. Chan, S. Chen, et al., "The red wine polyphenol resveratrol displays bilevel inhibition on aromatase in breast cancer cells," *Toxicological Sciences* 92 (1) (July 2006): 71–77.

4. R. H. Dashwood, "Frontiers in polyphenols and cancer prevention," *Journal of Nutrition* 137 (1 supplement) (January 2007): 267S–269S.

5. G. G. Duthie, P. T. Gardner, and J. A. Kyle, "Plant polyphenols: are they the new magic bullet?" *Proceedings of the Nutrition Society* 62 (3) (August 2003): 599–603.

6. R. L. Galli, B. Shukitt-Hale, K. A. Youdim, and J. A. Joseph, "Fruit polyphenolics and brain aging: nutritional interventions targeting age-related neuronal and behavioral deficits," *Annals of the New York Academy of Sciences* 959 (April 2002): 128–132.

7. B. D. Gehm, J. M. McAndrews, P. Y. Chien, and J. L. Jameson, "Resveratrol, a polyphenolic compound found in grapes and wine, is an agonist for the estrogen receptor," *Proceedings of the National Academy of Sciences of the United States of America* 94 (25) (December 1997): 14138–14143.

8. D. M. Goldberg, J. Yan, and G. J. Soleas, "Absorption of three wine-related polyphenols in three different matrices by healthy subjects," *Chemical Biochemistry* 36 (1) (February 2003): 79–87.

9. J. Leikert, T. Rathel, P. Wohlfart, V. Cheynier, et al., "Red wine polyphenols enhance endothelial nitric oxide synthase expression and subsequent nitric oxide release from endothelial cells," *Circulation* 106 (13) (September 24, 2002): 1614–1617.

10. C. Manach, A. Scalbert, C. Morand, C. Rémésy, et al., "Polyphenols: food sources and bioavailability," *American Journal of Clinical Nutrition* 79 (5) (May 2004): 727–747.

11. J. Martinez and J. J. Moreno, "Effect of resveratrol, a natural polyphenolic compound, on reactive oxygen species and prostaglandin production," *Biochemical Pharmacology* 59 (7) (April 1, 2000): 865–870.

12. S. Quideau, "Plant 'polyphenolic' small molecules can induce a calorie restriction mimetic life-span extension by activating sirtuins: will 'polyphenols' someday be used as chemotherapeutic drugs in Western medicine?" *Chembiochem* 5 (4) (April 2, 2004): 427–430.

13. A. Scalbert, I. T. Johnson, and M. Saltmarsh, "Polyphenols: antioxidants and beyond," *American Journal of Clinical Nutrition* 81 (1 supplement) (January 2005): 215S–217S.

14. N. Wade, "Red wine ingredient increases endurance, study shows," *New York Times*, November 17, 2006.

15. T. Wallerath. G. Deckert, T. Ternes, H. Anderson, et al., "Resveratrol, a polyphenolic phytoalexin present in red wine, enhances expression and activity of endothelial nitric oxide synthase," *Circulation* 106 (13) (September 24, 2002): 1652–1658.

16. J. M. Wu, Z. R. Wang, T. C. Hsih, J. L. Bruder, et al., "Mechanism of cardioprotection by resveratrol, a phenolic antioxidant present in red wine (review)," *International Journal of Molecular Medicine* 8 (1) (July 2001) 3–17.

17. N. Al-Awwadi, J. Axay, P. Poucheret, G. Cassanas, et al., "Antidiabetic activity of red wine polyphenolic extract, ethanol, or both in streptozotocintreated rats," *Journal of Agricultural and Food Chemistry* 52 (4) (February 25, 2004): 1008–1016.

18. A. A. Bertelli, M. Migliori, V. Panichi, N. Origlia, et al., "Resveratrol, a component of wine and grapes, in the prevention of kidney disease," *Annals of the New York Academy of Sciences* 957 (May 2002): 230–238.

19. A. A. Bertelli, L. Giovanni, R. Stradi, S. Urien, et al., "Kinetics of trans- and cis-resveratrol (3, 4', 5-trihydroxstilbene) after red wine oral administration in rats," *International Journal of Clinical Pharmacology Research* 16 (4–5) (1996): 77–81.

20. A. A. Bertelli, L. Giovanni, R. Stradi, J. P. Tillement, et al., "Plasma, urine and tissue levels of trans- and cis-resveratrol (3,4',5-trihydroxystilbene) after short-term or prolonged administration of red wine to rats," *International Journal of Tissue Reactions* 18 (2–3) (1996): 67–71.

21. G. Cao and R. L. Prior, "Red wine in moderation: potential health benefits independent of alcohol," *Nutrition in Clinical Care* 3 (2) (March–April 2000): 76–82.

22. M. A. Carluccio, L. Siculella, M. A. Ancora, M. Massaro, et al., "Olive oil and red wine antioxidant polyphenols inhibit endothelial activation: antiatherogenic properties of Mediterranean diet phytochemicals," *Arteriosclerosis, Thrombosis, and Vascular Biology* 23 (4) (April 1, 2003): 622–629.

23. R. Corder, J. A. Douthwaite, D. M. Lees, N. Q. Khan, et al., "Endothelin-1 synthesis reduced by red wine," *Nature* 414 (6866) (December 20–27, 2001): 863–864.

24. R. Corder, W. Mullen, N. Q. Khan, S. C. Marks, et al., "Oenology: red wine procyanidins and vascular health," *Nature* 444 (7119) (November 30, 2006): 566.

25. A. Cordova, L. Jackson, D. Berke-Schlessel, and B. Sumpio. "The cardio-vascular protective effect of red wine," *Journal of the American College of Surgeons* 200 (3) (March 2005): 428–439.

26. C. de Santi, A. Pietrabissa, F. Mosca, and G. M. Pacifici, "Glucuronidation of resveratrol, a natural product present in grape and wine, in the human liver," *Xenobiotica* 30 (11) (November 2000): 1047–1054.

27. C. de Santi, A. Pietrabissa, R. Spisni, F. Mosca, et al., "Sulphation of resveratrol, a natural product present in grapes and wine, in the human liver and duodenum," *Xenobiotica* 30 (6) (June 2000): 609–617.

28. J. Dudley and D. Das, "Resveratrol, a polyphenolic antioxidant in red wine, is dose-dependent in delivering cardioprotection," *Experimental Biology* 2007: meeting abstracts 114.5.

29. E. N. Frankel, J. Kanner, J. B. German, E. Parks, et al., "Inhibition of oxidation of human low-density lipoprotein by phenolic substances in red wine," *Lancet* 341 (8843) (February 20, 1993): 454–457.

30. B. Fuhrman, A. Lavy, and M. Aviram, "Consumption of red wine with meals reduces the susceptibility of human plasma and low-density lipoprotein to lipid peroxidation," *American Journal of Clinical Nutrition* 61 (3) (March 1995) 549–554.

31. J. B. German and R. L. Walzem, "The health benefits of wine," *Annual Review of Nutrition* 20 (2000): 561–593.

32. D. M. Goldberg, J. Yan, E. Ng, E. P. Diamandis, et al., "A global survey of *trans*-resveratrol concentrations in commercial wines," *American Journal of Enology and Viticulture* 46 (2) (1995): 159–165.

33. A. L. Klatsky, G. D. Friedman, M. A. Armstrong, and H. Kipp, "Wine, liquor, beer, and mortality," *American Journal of Epidemiology* 158 (6) (September 15, 2003): 585–595.

34. P. Kopp, "Resveratrol, a phytoestrogen found in red wine: a possible explanation for the conundrum of the 'French paradox?' " *European Journal of Endocrinology* 138 (6) (June 1998): 619–620.

35. D. Leibovici, K. Ritchie, B. Ledésert, and J. Touchon, "The effects of wine and tobacco consumption on cognitive performance in the elderly: a longitudinal study of relative risk," *International Journal of Epidemiology* 28 (1) (February 1999): 77–81.

36. M. López-Vélez, F. Martínez-Martínez, and C. Del Valle-Ribes, "The study of phenolic compounds as natural antioxidants in wine," *Critical Reviews in Food Science and Nutrition* 43 (3) (2003): 233–244.

37. M. Maggiolini, A. G. Recchia, D. Bonofiglio, S. Cantalano, et al., "The red wine phenolics piceatannol and myricetin act as agonists for estrogen receptor in human breast cancer cells," *Journal of Molecular Endocrinology* 35 (2) (October 2005): 269–281.

38. J. F. Moreno-Labanda, R. Mallavia, L. Pérez-Fons, V. Lizama, et al., "Deter-

mination of piceid and resveratrol in Spanish wines deriving from *Monastrell (Vitis vinifera L.)* grape variety," *Journal of Agricultural and Food Chemistry* 52 (17) (August 25, 2004): 5396–5403.

39. F. Orallo, E. Alvarez, M. Camiña, J. M. Leiro, et al., "The possible implication of trans-resveratrol in the cardioprotective effects of long-term moderate wine consumption," *Molecular Pharmacology* 61 (2) (February 2002): 294–302.

40. J. Orgogozo, J. F. Dartigues, S. Lafont, L. Letenneur, et al., "Wine consumption and dementia in the elderly: a prospective community study in the Bordeaux area," *Revue Neurologique* 153 (3) (April 1997): 185–192.

41. C. R. Pace-Asciak, O. Rounova, S. E. Hahn, E. P. Diamandis, et al. "Wines and grape juices as modulators of platelet aggregation in healthy human subjects," *Clinica Chimica Acta* 246 1996 (1–2) (March 15, 1996): 163–182.

42. E. B Rimm, A. Klatsky, D. Grobbee, and M. J. Stampfer, "Review of moderate alcohol consumption and reduced risk of coronary heart disease: is the effect due to beer, wine, or spirits?" *British Medical Journal* 312 (7033) (March 23, 1996): 731–736.

43. A. I. Romero-Pérez, R. M. Lamuela-Raventós, A. L. Waterhouse, and M. C. de la Torre-Boronat, "Levels of *cis-* and *trans*-resveratrol and their glucosides in white and rosé *Vitis vinifera* wines from Spain," *Journal of Agriculture and Food Chemistry* 44 (8) (1996): 2124–2128.

44. H. H. Siemann and L. L. Creasy, "Concentration of the phytoalexin resveratrol in wine," *American Journal of Enology and Viticulture* 43 (1) (1992): 49–52.

45. D. Stipp, "So what's the scoop on that stuff in red wine that's supposed to let you live forever?" *Fortune,* February 5, 2007.

46. J. F. Tomera, "Current knowledge of the health benefits and disadvantages of wine consumption," *Trends in Food Science and Technology* 10 (4–5) (April 1999): 129–138.

47. G. J. Soleas, E. P. Diamandis, and D. M. Goldberg, "Wine as a biological fluid: history, production, and role in disease prevention," *Journal of Clinical Laboratory Analysis* 11 (5) (1997): 287–313.

48. D. M. Goldberg, S. E. Hahn, and J. G. Parkes: "Beyond alcohol: beverage consumption and cardiovascular mortality," *Clinica Chimica Acta* 237 (1–2) (June 15, 1995): 155–187.

49. W. B. Kannel and R. C. Ellison, "Alcohol and coronary heart disease: the evidence for a protective effect," *Clinica Chimica Acta* 246 (1–2) (March 15, 1996): 59–76.

50. P. Galet: *A practical ampelography, grapevine identification,* 2nd ed. (Ithaca, NY: Comstock Publishing Company, 1980).

51. D. D. Crippen Jr. and J. C. Morrison, "The effects of sun exposure on the phenolic content of Cabernet Sauvignon berries during development," *American Journal of Enology and Viticulture* 37 (4) (1986): 243–247.

52. K. Hahlbrock, "Flavonoids," in *The biochemistry of plants,* vol. 7, P. K. Stumpf and E. E. Conn, eds. (New York: Academic Press, 1981).

53. W. Bors and M. Saran, "Radical scavenging by flavonoid antioxidants," *Free Radical Research Communications* 2 (4–6) (1987): 289–294.

54. P. L. Teissedre, E. N. Frankel, A. L. Waterhouse, H. Peleg, et al., "Inhibition of in vitro human LDL oxidation by phenolic antioxidants from grapes and wines," *Journal of the Science of Food and Agriculture* 70 (1) (1996): 55–61.

55. G. Kaur, L. V. Rao, A. Agrawal, and U. R. Pendurthi, "Effect of wine phenolics on cytokine-induced C-reactive protein expression," *Journal of Thrombosis and Haemostasis* 5 (6) (June 2007): 1309–1317.

56. S. Sutcliffe, E. Giovannucci, M. F. Leitzmann, E. B Rimm, et al., "A prospective cohort study of red wine consumption and risk of prostate cancer," *International Journal of Cancer* 120 (7) (April 1, 2007): 1529–1535.

57. C. A. de la Lastra and I. Villegas, "Resveratrol as an anti-inflammatory and anti-aging agent: mechanisms and clinical implications," *Molecular Nutrition and Food Research* 49 (5) (May 2005): 405–430.

58. N. Elmali, O. Baysal, A. Harma, I. Esenkaya, et al., "Effects of resveratrol in inflammatory arthritis," *Inflammation* 30 (1–2) (April 2007): 1–6.

59. O. Ates, S. Cayli, E. Altinoz, I. Gurses, et al., "Neuroprotection by resveratrol against traumatic brain injury in rats," *Molecular and Cellular Biochemistry* 294 (1–2) (January 2007): 137–144.

60. F. Bianchini and H. Vainio, "Wine and resveratrol: mechanisms of cancer prevention?," *European Journal of Cancer Prevention* 12 (5) (October 2003): 417–425.

61. A. Damianaki, E. Bakogeorgou, M. Kampa, G. Notas, et al., "Potent inhibitory action of red wine polyphenols on human breast cancer cells," *Journal of Cellular Biochemistry* 78 (3) (June 6, 2000): 429–441.

62. L. J. Fooks and G. R. Gibson. "Probiotics as modulators of the gut flora," *British Journal of Nutrition* 88 (2002): s39–s49.

CHAPTER 19: THE FOUR-STEP XENO LONGEVITY WEIGHT-LOSS PROGRAM

1. J. W. Anderson, E. C. Konz, R. C. Frederich, and C. L. Wood, "Long-term weight-loss maintenance: a meta-analysis of US studies," *American Journal of Clinical Nutrition* 74 (5) (November 2001): 579–584.

2. P. M. Ridker, "High-sensitivity C-reactive protein, potential adjunct for global risk assessment in the primary prevention of cardiovascular disease," *Circulation* 103 (13) (April 3, 2001): 1813–1818.
3. ImPACT concussion testing, www.impacttest.com, accessed July 31, 2008.
4. M. Rosenbaum, J. Hirsch, E. Murphy, and R. L. Leibel, "Effects of changes in body weight on carbohydrate metabolism, catecholamine excretion, and thyroid function," *American Journal of Clinical Nutrition* 71 (6) (June 2000): 1421–1432.
5. J. A. Banzer, T. E. Maguire, C. M. Kennedy, C. J. O'Malley, et al., "Results of cardiac rehabilitation in patients with diabetes mellitus," *American Journal of Cardiology* 93 (1) (January 1, 2004): 81–84.
6. Joseph C. Maroon and Jeffrey Bost, *Fish oil: the natural anti-inflammatory* (Laguna Beach, CA: Basic Health Publications, 2006).
7. J. C. Maroon, "Presidential address: from Aequanimitas to Icarus," *Clinical Neurosurgery* 34 (1988): 3–15.
8. William H. Danforth, *I dare you* (St. Louis: Kessinger Publishing, 1941).
9. J. M. Schwartz and S. Begley, *The mind and the brain: neuroplasticity and the power of mental force* (New York: ReganBooks, 2002).
10. P. J. Rogers and H. J. Smit, "Food craving and food 'addiction': a critical review of the evidence from a biopsychosocial perspective," *Pharmacology Biochemistry and Behavior* 66 (1) (May 2000): 3–14.
11. Viktor E. Frankl, *Man's search for meaning* (Boston: Beacon Press, 1959).
12. Mihaly Csikszentmihalyi, *Flow: the psychology of optimal experience* (New York: Harper and Row, 1990).
13. K. Ellison, "Mastering your own mind," *Psychology Today,* September–October 2006.
14. K. M. Sancier and D. Holman, "Multifaceted health benefits of medical qigong," *Journal of Alternative and Complementary Medicine* 10 (1) (2004): 163–166.
15. C. Kummer, "Your genomic diet: our genetic profile could be the key to staying healthy and eating right," *Technology Review,* August 2005.
16. D. Della Penna, "Review nutritional genomics: manipulating plant micronutrients to improve human health," *Science* 285 (5426) (July 16, 1999): 375–379.
17. S. B. Eaton, M. Konner, and M. Shostak, "Stone agers in the fast lane: chronic degenerative diseases in evolutionary perspective," *American Journal of Medicine* 84 (4) (April 1988): 739–749.
18. S. B. Eaton, "Humans, lipids and evolution," *Lipids* 27 (10) (October 1992): 814–820.

19. S. B. Eaton, S. B. Eaton III, and M. J. Konner, "Paleolithic nutrition revisited: a twelve year retrospective on its nature and implications," *European Journal of Clinical Nutrition* 51 (4) (April 1997): 207–216.

20. S. B. Eaton, S. B. Eaton III, A. J. Sinclair, L. Cordain, et al., "Dietary intake of long chain polyunsaturated fatty acids during the Paleolithic," *World Review of Nutrition and Dietetics* 83 (1998): 12–23.

21. Michael F. Roizen and Mehmet C. Oz, *You: Staying Young* (New York: Simon & Schuster, 2007).

22. C. Manach, A. Scalbert, C. Morand, C. Rémésy, et al., "Polyphenols: food sources and bioavailability," *American Journal of Clinical Nutrition* 79 (5) (May 2004): 727–747.

23. Centers for Disease Control and Prevention (CDC): www.fruitsand veggiesmatter.gov.

24. Sanjay Gupta, *Chasing life: new discoveries in the search for immortality to help you age less today* (New York: Warner Wellness, 2007).

CHAPTER 20: SUMMING UP

1. W. Somerset Maugham, *The Summing Up* (New York: Vintage Classics, 1938).

2. Charles Dickens, *A Tale of Two Cities* (London: Chapman and Hall, 1859).

3. Dylan Thomas, "Do not go gentle into that good night," 1951.

4. R. Weindruch and S. R. Spindler, "Lifespan project launched: the goal: to find practical methods of retarding the aging process," *Life Extension,* August 1997.

5. Thomas T. Perls and Margery Hutter Silver, with John F. Lauerman, *Living to 100* (New York: Basic Books, 1999).

6. D. A. Sinclair, "Toward a unified theory of caloric restriction and longevity regulation," *Mechanisms of Ageing and Development* 126 (9) (September 2005): 987–1002.

7. James R. Carey and Shripad Tuljapurkar, *Life span: evolutionary, ecological and demographic perspectives* (New York: Population Council, 2003).

8. J. R. Wilmoth, L. J. Deegan, H. Lundström, and S. Horiuchi, "Increase of maximum life-span in Sweden, 1861–1999," *Science* 289 (5488) (September 29, 2000): 2366–2368.

9. Employee Benefit Research Institute, www.ebri.org, accessed July 31, 2008.

10. International Union for the Scientific Study of Population, www.iussp .org, accessed July 31, 2008.

11. J. M. Robine and K. Ritchie, "Healthy life expectancy: evaluation of global

indicator of change in population health," *British Medical Journal* 302 (6774) (February 23, 1991): 457–460.

12. E. A. Schoenhofen, D. F. Wyszynski, S. Andersen, J. Pennington, et al., "Characteristics of 32 supercentenarians," *Journal of the American Geriatrics Society* 54 (8) (August 2006): 1237–1240.

13. T. T. Perls, I. V. Kohler, S. Andersen, E. Schoenhofen, et al., "Survival of parents and siblings of supercentenarians," *Journals of Gerontology Series A: Biological Sciences and Medical Sciences* 62A (9) (September 1, 2007): 1028–1034.

Index

NOTE: Bold numbers refer to figure and picture captions.